THE LAST FITNESS BOOK
YOU WILL EVER NEED

GET FIT!

THE LAST FITNESS BOOK

YOU WILL EVER NEED

GET FIT!

LARRY NORTH

THE SUMMIT GROUP

THE SUMMIT GROUP

1227 West Magnolia, Suite 500, Fort Worth, Texas 76104

The suggestions for food, stretching, exercise, weight training and all other health-and-fitness related subjects in this book are not intended as a substitute for consultation with your nutritionist, fitness instructor and/or physician. Before starting any aspect of the North Program, you are advised to consult your physician or a qualified health professional for specific guidance. The use of specific products in this book does not constitute an endorsement by the authors or the publisher.

Publisher's Cataloging in Publication
(Prepared by Quality Books, Inc.)

North, Larry.
    Get Fit! : the last fitness book you will ever need / Larry North
    p. cm.
    ISBN 1-56530-026-2

    1. Physical fitness.   2. Health.   3. Nutrition.   I. Title

RA781.N67 1993   613.7
                                          QB193-1014

To My Family

FOREWORD

As a syndicated sports columnist and author in Dallas, I've developed a reputation for doing my homework and telling the truth. No hero worship. No hidden agendas. No fear of how star athletes or legendary coaches will treat me if I write fairly and honestly about how they really are.

Above all I value my integrity.

So please believe that I believe in this book and how it can change your life.

One other thing about me: Fitness is my passion. I had run ten marathons and had been lifting weights for ten years before I met Larry North. I had studied food, and how and when to eat it almost as intensely as I've followed the Dallas Cowboys. So I knew enough to know whether Larry was just another fitness-fad fraud, telling you what you want to hear instead of what you need to know.

Larry North has humbled me with his knowledge. I waited to catch him in a half-truth or inconsistency. He passed my test.

I learned more about weight training in one one-hour session with Larry than I had from eight or ten instructors I've known for ten years. Even now, I can't listen to Larry's KLIF radio show without picking up new fat-free nuggets. Larry amazes me with his range—his expertise in all fitness fields. He combines the easy-to-digest best of a nutritionist, a dietitian, a bodybuilder, a power lifter,

a martial-arts instructor, an aerobics teacher, a fitness counselor—
and your best friend.

Larry is a rare expert in all those areas, and he's pretty good
about talking about life, too. Larry survived a tough childhood.
Larry is no high-and-mighty, out-of-touch professor. He's smart
and street-smart. He has uncommon common sense. He doesn't
talk down to you. He talks to you, in your language.

Nothing in this book is sugarcoated, including the recommended foods. Larry very simply tells you the truth about how to
make your body look and feel better, forever. His principles are
sound. They will endure. This book will not be obsolete in six
months.

Just as important, these words are aimed at real people living
real lives. Nonstop lives in restaurants and hotels. Stress-filled lives
in a society fraught with tasty temptation. What to eat, and when?
When to work out, and how? You're about to find out, once and for
all, from a man who lives the same hectic life you do.

Trust me, Larry North knows.

— *Skip Bayless*

ACKNOWLEDGMENTS

This book could not have happened without the contributions of so many people. Their insights gave this book the kind of depth and power that I could not have contributed alone. I want to thank each member of my staff working with me at Larry North Total Fitness, my gym in Dallas, Texas, especially Nancy Todd. My rise would not have been possible without Dan Bennett and Dallas radio station KLIF. Thank you for taking a chance on me in 1989 by asking me to host the "Weekend Workout," a health and fitness talk show.

I want to thank Cliff Sheats for the countless hours of conversation we've had about food and nutrition. I also want to express my gratitude to Houston nutrition wizard Keith Klein for sharing his knowledge about all aspects of health and fitness, and to Joey Antonio, Ph.D., who provided a critical analysis of the scientific aspects of this book. And maybe the person who has had the most influence on me is Melanie Peskett. Not only did she come up with all of the recipes mentioned in this book, and not only does she make the best low-fat food I have ever tasted, she also has been the heart and soul of my motivation to accomplish so many of my goals. Also, a special heartfelt thanks go out to the Mauros, my surrogate family.

Thanks to my literary agent Jan Miller and associate agent David Smith for overseeing the creation of this book. Years ago, Jan was the first person I ever trained professionally, and even then she was telling me I needed to write a book. Truly, she is the one who discovered me. Thanks to Shannon Peterson and Skip Hollandsworth for help in writing this manuscript. Thanks to Skip Bayless, the world's greatest sportswriter, for contributing his comments and the foreword. And I want to thank The Summit Group publishing company for making this book possible, especially Mark Hulme, Brent Lockhart, Mike Towle, Cheryl Corbitt and Joe Bishop.

It's hard to name all of the friends who have helped me. But I must thank David MacDonald, Pat Beaird, Steve Bloomberg and Doug Murphy for their encouragement. Others made great contributions to the book: Jim and Gayle Ziaks Halperin, Steve Ivy, David Hall and Andrew Tobias. I thank the dozens of restaurants that put "The North Plate" on their menus. And I would like to especially thank the staff of the Texas Council on Compulsive Gambling.

Finally, I must thank again my family—Mom, Adam, Alan and Dad. I will never forget the words of my father who was suffering from terminal cancer as I wrote this book. He said, "Larry, life at its best is a struggle and life at its longest is still short. So Larry, boy, don't do like your father, but take care of your health and remember your Daddy always loves you."

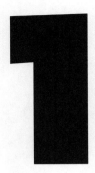

First, a Question

How Did You Get So
Messed Up About Food and Fitness?

know who you are. You've either never bought a diet or fitness book because you think they're bunk, or you've already got a stack of them in your closet. You have one that tells you to eat nothing but fruit. Another tells you to eat anything but carbohydrates. There's a book telling you the secret is in running marathons. There's one telling you to drink coffee before your workout so you'll burn off more fat. You're the type of person who turns on the television and feels guilty after watching one of those tennis shoe commercials that tell you to work out until you drop. Or you get tempted into buying some $19.95 contraption that fits between your thighs.

Oh, yeah, I know who you are. I have you come through my gym. Thousands of you have called in to my radio show. Utterly frustrated, you tell me that one week you're on the Pritikin diet, the next week you're with Dr. Atkins, the next week you're visiting Jenny Craig. One week you're able to lose ten pounds and fit into your jeans. The next week you've yo-yoed up ten pounds and you're back to wearing oversized shirts.

Someone tells you to eat more grapefruit because it will actually melt the fat away. You're off to the grocery store to buy a case of grapefruit. Someone else tells you the only exercise worth anything is exercise that makes you sweat. Off you go to the sporting goods store to buy a heavy sweat suit. If I told you that low-fat Alpo dog food would help you lose weight, I'm sure some of you would serve it for dinner. If you're honest, you'll admit you have no idea what you're supposed to do to develop a great body.

After eating a greasy hamburger, some of you figure that you only have to work out an extra hour and—presto!—you'll take care of that extra hamburger fat. Some of you think you can just peel the crust off fried chicken and have a healthy meal. Some of you, of course, are like PhD. nutritionists who know the number of calories that are in every bite of food. And you know what? You're still gaining weight!

Here we are nearing the twenty-first century and we are surrounded by more so-called diet and exercise experts than ever before. We are weight conscious to a degree that is without precedent in human history. And people are still worse off than ever before. At this moment, approximately half of the women and a quarter of the men in this country say they are on a diet to lose weight. Government reports tell us we're all trying to eat fewer calories. Yet in the end, those same statistics show that those people who diet are more likely to regain the pounds they shed— and then gain a few more!

We are still confounded by fat. Those of us between the ages of twenty and fifty are gaining an average of one to two pounds a year. The average weight of an American woman under the age of thirty is seven pounds heavier than her counterpart in 1959. My favorite statistic: The American Seating Company has announced that the fannies of Americans have widened by more than two inches in the last thirty years.

The Deception

How did this happen? Why, when we are flooded with gyms and diet gurus and aerobic instructors, are we failing to get fit as a country? Is it because we're just lazy? That we don't really try hard enough? That we're just a bunch of gluttonous Americans?

Is it because we have failed our fitness programs?

Or is it because our programs have failed us?

Before we go any further in this book, I want you to get one thing straight. You have not failed. There are times when I get absolutely livid thinking about what has happened to you. I think about how you've been subjected to the claims of those weight-loss programs that say they are "medically supervised" and then ask you to starve yourself of vital nutrients. Or I see these authors talking about their "guaranteed plan" to dieting. I've taken a look at these companies promising you a new body with the latest "revolutionary diet foods." It makes me want to throw up. If you've tried some of these diets, you've probably found yourself wanting to do the same thing.

Please, please, don't blame yourself. You're having to deal with everyone from charlatans making promises that cannot be kept to well-intentioned health professionals who still are trying to pass on very misguided fitness programs.

It breaks my heart to watch how hard many of you try. I know about you overweight men and women who eat less—less!—than all your co-workers you lunch with from the office. I know how great your willpower has been, how courageous and dedicated you've been to dieting.

I know about your long, dismal history of trying to lose weight— the changes, the turnarounds, the gains and losses. I know you have never eaten a dessert without feeling guilty. I know there are times, after an entire day of being "good," when you find yourself late at night eating by yourself. I know how you beat your brains out at aerobics classes until your ankles are swollen and your knees stiff. And I know what it does to you when you don't get or stay any thinner.

I know all about this, you see, because I grew up in such a world. My mother spent most of her life obsessed about losing weight. She would starve all week, take amphetamines ("diet pills," she called them), and then find herself bingeing all through the weekend. She got so addicted to diet pills that she needed them not to lose weight, but just to stay awake through the day.

My mother went for weeks eating nothing but hard-boiled eggs and cottage cheese. She was in the very first Overeaters Anonymous chapter in the country. She joined Weight Watchers. She would send off for every weight-loss program advertised in the back of magazines. After trying the Beverly Hills Diet, she went around for days with her lips puckered due to eating all the pineapples that are recommended for that program. She tried diuretics and laxatives. She wore rubber gloves when preparing food because she was told that fat from meat could get into her pores and prevent her from losing weight.

I felt like I was in a madhouse. One afternoon when I was a boy, I was out with my mother, and I bought a hot dog with my carefully earned money. My mother was on one of her typical 500-calories-a-day diets. I hadn't even taken a bite of the hot dog and she shouted, "Look, Larry, over there! There's your father!" As I turned around, my mother grabbed the hot dog and stuck the whole thing in her mouth. The whole thing! I started crying—and so did my Mom. She was crying for what this absurd life of dieting had done to her—a life that would drive her to steal her own child's food.

When people ask me why I'm in this business, I repeat that story. I know there are many of you who sit alone and cry because you are so devastated about what's happened to your bodies. I know a lot of you are depressed with your lots in life, thinking you are now far too overweight to slim down or too flabby to ever get in shape.

And I want to tell you, just as I've told my mother, "You aren't the failure. You aren't the loser. No one could make a sacrifice like you. It's just that no one ever told you how to do the right program."

The North Program

So get ready. I have spent my life preparing for this book, preparing to bust the myths that have misled you for so long about what must be done to get a tight stomach and sleek hips and firmly toned muscles. It's time for a common-sense program that, in the end, is going to make you feel far more exhilarated and successful than anything you've ever tried before.

In the past, you have tried things that have put your body in an artificial state of deprivation. Now, I'm going to give you a program that is exactly the opposite—and permanent.

I say this almost every week on my radio show and I'll say it again: Any program that you can't do for the rest of your life is not worth doing for a single day.

With the North Program, you don't get shortcuts or secret formulas. You won't hear about any promises about your body changing overnight. But hasn't that always been the problem before? Instead of looking for quick answers, a "ten-easy-steps-to-fitness" plan, you need a program that works for life. One that isn't going to make you suffer through a self-destructive diet. One that can make working out fun again. That's what I've got.

Are You Skeptical?

Considering everything I've said already, you'd be a fool if you were not thinking, What can Larry North tell me that already hasn't been said a thousand times before? What am I setting myself up for, another babbling personal trainer?

I'm thrilled you're asking those questions, and I don't want you to stop asking them. In this book, I'll even ask many of the questions for you. You need to remain skeptical, because you've been manipulated for so long.

Believe me, you're not going to be reading one of these how-to books written by a Hollywood celebrity who has hours of free time each day to train. This isn't one of those books from someone who was once a world-famous athlete and believes you should work out like he once worked out. I'm not a quack medical doctor who's going to promise you a weight loss of five pounds a week. I am not going to give you all that big-time bodybuilding jargon ("Hey, guys, let's get ripped!"). Nor am I going to fill the book with pages of in-depth nutritional science information that you'll forget anyway. I won't do any of those things. But I do know who you are—the frustrated American who is just not sure how to get inspired, and certainly doesn't know what to do.

All I'm asking is that you give yourself one more chance. This time, you won't learn to be artificially thin. You'll learn to get lean. You will strip off fat. You will take your floppy bellies and mayon-naise-like thighs and sagging hips and you can re-create yourself. You will build sleekly defined muscles. You'll rediscover the sexy curves in your body. You will put a new energy and power into your life that will flabbergast your friends and family.

All I ask is that you wipe out all your old twisted notions of what diet and fitness is. Just think about it. You've already learned how to diet. Now let me teach you how to eat. You've learned how to do an aerobics class. Now I'm going to teach you the meaning of real aerobics. And you've probably experienced a terrifying day in the gym where you got sore straining under some weights. Now let me teach you the essence of real weight training, the kind that will make you, for the first time in your life, excited about the weight room, not dreading it as a Medieval torture chamber.

You Can Do This

I'll be honest. The North Program you're about to learn is nothing new. I didn't invent any of the things I'm going to be telling you. But I know that most of you have heard this only in little bits and pieces in the past. For the first time, you're going to get the whole program laid out for you in one book. If you care about reshaping your body, and you read this book, then you'll start seeing results. Even if you care about your body *just a little bit*, you'll see results.

The North Program is not a pass-or-fail program. If you want to get as lean as quickly as possible, then you can follow this program to the letter of the law and your body will transform itself. If you are forty years old and haven't worked out in years and have twenty extra pounds in your midsection, then you can start slower. In fact, you will never have to do 100 percent of this program—and your body will still go through a significant change. But I bet you that once you get into this, you'll want to follow it every day for the rest of your life.

Just be patient with me. The North Program—like anything that's important—is going to take a little time and concentration. It's going to take some motivation. But I will help you find that spot in yourself which demands excellence.

This is going to be fun. I wish I had the ability to express what it feels like to watch people get on the program and realize that they are enjoying themselves. They enjoy eating the right foods. They enjoy working out.

I want you too to get fired up for change. The past is behind you. When you finish this book, you're going to say, "Thank God, I've finally got it."

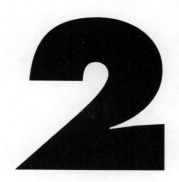

The "M" Word

The Key to
Your New Body

Don't panic. I'm about to say the "M" word out loud here, and I don't want you to start hyperventilating. I don't want you to think that I'm going to try to turn you into the next Arnold Schwarzenegger.

No, a thousand times no. My goal is not to turn you into one of those Neanderthal, vein-popping men or women you see pictured in magazines. But ladies and gentlemen, the key to the North Program—as it should be to any honest eating-and-fitness program—is the following word: Muscle.

I am talking here about muscle in its purest, most beautiful form. Not the big pumped-up muscle that wins bodybuilding shows. But the toned, well-fueled muscle that can change your body in myriad ways you don't even know about.

Incredibly, this is the great taboo subject in the field of diet and exercise. So many other writers are scared to death that if they mention muscles, they aren't going to sell any books. If you read their diet books with the obligatory little chapter in the back reminding you to get in some "exercise," you're going to fail, I promise you. You're being led down another rabbit trail. You're not getting the message that I am going to tell you up front, loud and clear: The great key to changing your body is to change your body's muscle. It's not dieting that will be your golden secret. It's not running enough so you can finish a marathon. It's muscle.

Please don't get caught up in that old muscle-head stereotype that for years has kept people from succeeding. Just for the next few paragraphs, let me explain a little basic science that few so-called experts ever try to tell you.

Your metabolism is everything your body does to convert nutrients into energy. Your metabolism, for example, maintains your body temperature. It controls your body's activities like breathing and the beating of your heart.

Here's the great little secret about metabolism: If you get your body to speed up its metabolism—to speed up the way it burns fuel—then you will have the major solution to being overweight. You'll be able to quickly burn off the food you eat and also burn the large reserves of fat cells in your body.

Despite all the reports and studies that have come out over the years about diet and food, and the human body, there is still one basic fact that can't be refuted: To lose weight, you have to burn more calories than you take in. To do that, you must have a great metabolism.

And to get a great metabolism, you've got to have—you guessed it!—muscle.

You can't ignore this one critical fact about the human body: Fat tissue in your body collects fat, and muscle tissue in your body burns fuel. Your muscles require more calories to function. Fat, however, is less metabolically active because its function is to serve as a big old greasy warehouse for the storage of fat cells.

You need to think of each muscle as a minifurnace. The more muscle you have, the more your body burns off fuel. And that's not when you are just exercising. Your resting metabolic rate will also be much higher if you increase the amount of muscle in your body.

The Essence of the Program

So, you have got to stop deceiving yourself about the next diet that's going to come around and start figuring out how to trigger your metabolism. That's the goal of the North Program. I'm going to teach you how to increase your metabolism by:

1. Putting you on an eating program—not a diet program—that will give you the right foods to increase your muscle and decrease your fat. Or, as I like to say, I want you to feed the muscle and starve the fat.

2. Getting you to eat that food spread out in small meals throughout the day, which, remarkably, makes your metabolism work even faster.

3. Teaching you how to increase your muscle because muscle is your best ally to losing weight. And that means one thing: weight training.

Okay, you're thinking, here it comes. I'm going to have to head to the gym for four hours a day.

Stop right there. The great myth in this business is that you have to strain and grunt to reshape your body. I am going to teach you about weight training, not weightlifting—body shaping, not bodybuilding. I'm going to ask you to use that three-pound "muscle" in your head—your brain. The North Program is not about who trains the hardest, but who trains the smartest.

As you'll find out in later chapters, by carefully and naturally building your muscles, you will not only increase your metabolism and burn fat. You will also start sculpting your body in a way that no diet or aerobics class can do for you. You will get beautifully and subtly defined muscles, extremely lean physiques. And, under the North Program, you won't have to punish yourself to get there.

The Inevitable Truth About Your Body

I'm going to hide nothing from you. You have got to commit yourself to a routine of weight training. You need to see the weight room as your own personal fountain of youth. The main reason we get fatter as we get older is that we lose our muscle tissue. As we get older, our body's metabolism naturally slows down by 2 to 3 percent a decade. The only way to fight it is to build more muscle. Moreover, listen to this, you women readers: Because you have less muscle, pound for pound, than men, you already have slower metabolisms. The fat is more readily stored than burned as energy. The only way to fight it is to build more muscle.

There is no quicker, better way to get leaner than by following this program. "Oh, right," you're saying, "here we go again with the same old promises." Let me tell you something. For a long time, even I refused to believe such a claim. I grew up with the same habits as my mother. I was a compulsive overeater. I had been put on diets since the third grade, when I was told only to eat salads and carrots. I was like a lab rat, given huge amounts of diet pills and cottage cheese.

If I ever got my weight down, I was so weak from hunger I could not play with other boys. I was humiliated on playgrounds and in sports. In high school, I couldn't lift the bar of the Universal bench press machine even when it had no weight at all on it.

Finally, I decided to do one of these Charles Atlas-like transformations with my flabby body. I began lifting weights maniacally. I was a monster in the weight room, going there twice a day, taking the bus or riding my bike when my car broke down.

I did eventually turn into a bodybuilder. I would starve myself for weeks before a bodybuilding contest just so it would look like I had no body fat. The minute the contest was over, my body fat once again soared skywards. And then I said, "Wait a minute. This is no way to live. There's got to be a better way than starving myself or living the rest of my life in the weight room."

So, instead of living on the extremes, I began to take from the best of the programs I knew—the right way to eat, the right way to work out—and I began to adapt it for everyone. Fitness and health became my goal, not dieting and contests. Remember this: I, too, know about the curse of the fat gram. If there's one thing I can't stand, it's listening to fitness philosophy from people who are so genetically gifted that they have never known what it means to struggle to get their bodies lean. But after a lot of disappointment, I have discovered the program that works. It is all about the glory of the muscle.

The Program for Everyone

I'm talking to everyone here—the teenager and the seventy-year-old grandfather. Someone with a birdlike appetite and someone who's always ravenous. Those who put on weight easily and those who have difficulty putting on weight no matter how much they eat. For all of you, the key is to stimulate the development of more muscle tissue.

This program is also for those of you who might weigh the same as you did when you were sixteen—but you know that your body has lost its shape. This is for those of you who have become masters at wearing the kind of clothing that lets you hide that last unwanted five or ten pounds. Deep down, you're wondering, What is it going to take to get a little bit leaner? This is for those of you who are even very athletic and already muscular, but who don't know yet what it means to be fit.

This program is for those of you still willing to make yourself starve until you look like a victim of world hunger, just so someone can come up to you and say, "Wow, you look great!" The truth is that behind your back, everyone is saying, "Wow, you look deprived!"

Why, my friends, do you want to go through one more typical diet and lose some weight, and still look only like a slightly smaller version of your old body? Why do you want to do one more diet that will turn you from a big-shaped pear into a smaller-shaped pear? What if you could reshape the pear with new muscle? You've got a chance to free yourself from the tyranny of the past. The North Program won't seem like a sacrifice, but a blessing.

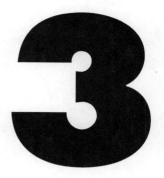

The Workout Myth

What True
Exercise Is — And Isn't

Why, if exercise is this one wonderful activity that can improve your health, are there so few of you out pounding the roads with your jogging feet or swimming laps in pools? Why, if exercise is renowned as the one great trump card you have to play in order to lose weight and reshape your body, do so few people regularly follow any exercise program at all? Why, especially, do few overweight people attempt even the most undemanding of exercises—such as walking?

According to the U.S. Department of Health, less than 10 percent of the population exercises three or more times a week to improve their fitness. And frankly, among that 10 percent I do see working out, few of you are doing it correctly.

I know exactly why most of you don't want to work out. Somewhere in your unconscious mind you still think of exercise as punishment. You remember the way you got taunted when you couldn't climb the rope in seventh grade P.E. class. You remember the humiliation of not passing that President's Council on Physical Fitness test. Even those of you who were once athletes remember those draining wind sprints and two-a-day workouts.

Sadly, there are a lot of you—most significantly you baby boomers who went through the aerobics class craze of the 1980s—who continue to believe only the most strenuous exercise has any impact on your life. You've been told by the Aerobics Mafia that the kind of exercise that's important is the type which pushes the body to the limits of endurance. If you aren't sweating profusely, you think, you're doing something wrong. With that kind of attitude prevalent in our society, it's no wonder overweight people don't even try to get in shape. They figure they will never catch up. They decide their nice jogging suit would best be used as an outfit to watch television in.

That Frightening Word—Aerobics

Well, here comes a dangerous confession. I hate the word "aerobics."

Don't get me wrong. It's not that I hate what aerobics truly means. It's that I hate what aerobics has come to stand for.

I go bonkers when someone tells me that aerobics means going for "the burn," as Jane Fonda and her followers exhort you to do on their exercise tapes. If that's what motivates you, that's fine. I'm all for it. But just because you are performing the "Super Fat Burning Aerobics Bench Class," don't think you're burning fat. And don't think you're gaining extra muscle just because your lungs are gasping for air and your leg muscles are burning. You're probably not gaining muscle.

I hope you're thinking, What? Has Larry lost his mind? He's speaking sacrilege in the fitness world. Surely, he's kidding.

I'm not kidding. I'm not one of these guys who is going to give you that old coach's speech about heavy, vein-popping exercise being the very thing that builds your character. Please, let's get rid of the Knute Rockne attitude. We're talking fitness here. We're not talking athletics. And that is a crucial difference.

Exercise—especially aerobic exercise—remains a widely misunderstood activity, which ultimately means it gets neglected in weight reduction. Let me go through some of the aerobic myths that are out there: So many of you believe (1) you need to sweat to lose weight, or (2) that you shouldn't eat before a workout so that your exercise will start right to work on your excess fat, or (3) that the longer you go without eating after exercise, the more fat is burned off, or (4) that you shouldn't drink any water while working out.

And then there are just as many myths about why you shouldn't work out. Some of you believe, for example, that if you exercise too much, your appetite will expand in gigantic proportions, canceling out the benefits of the exercise.

No. The truth is that the more sedentary you become, the more your appetite is increased, not decreased. You might have heard it said that the reason cattle farmers put their cows in pens and feed them is because they know the inactivity among the cattle will lead to lots of fat, and thus create more tender steaks.

What Is a True Workout?

Now I want you to listen to me very carefully. I know you're out there dieting and trying to eat right. But I also know you're not making a similar commitment to exercise.

You are willing to accept obesity, bad blood circulation, shortened breath, and all of those minor aches and pains that you could get rid of simply by working out. You remain listless because you don't work out. If you're thinking that exercise deprives you of energy, then you are the victim of another myth. The right kind of exercise boosts your body's ability to take in oxygen and to use it in making new energy.

There are so many scientific studies that continue to prove that exercise is the piece of the puzzle that's missing from most people's lives. In one study involving seventy-five women, twenty-five of them dieted only, twenty-five women exercised only, and twenty-five women did a combination of diet and exercise. Every woman who lost weight as a result of diet alone lost less fat and more muscle than the women who exercised. Conclusion: if you want to lose body fat, you must exercise.

Just as some of you work out all the time and aren't healthy because you refuse to eat right, there are far more of you who never get fit even though you eat right because you don't know how to exercise.

But being in shape doesn't have anything to do with being a good performer in an aerobics class or on a basketball court. It's as different as night and day. The way to cut fat out of the body is not to exercise as quickly as possible and as hard as possible. It is not doing things that leave you open-mouthed with exhaustion, your face feverish, your body barely able to stand.

In an upcoming chapter, you are going to get a program of true aerobics—the kind that knocks the fat off your body. We now know that to lose weight, we need to use the kind of aerobics that are low in intensity and long in duration. When you keep your entire body in motion for a very long period of time—and when you don't over-exert yourself—you're going to burn off your fat. Believe it. The more time you spend exercising at a solid, comfortable pace, the more you hit your fat stores.

This should be shocking and tremendous news for those of you still stuck thinking of aerobics as an intense sporting activity. People who think of me as the big athletic muscle man are always stunned when I tell them what I do for aerobics. Three to four times a week, I walk. That's right. And I know I am burning fat.

So How Do You Propose to Change My Body?

One of the great mistakes many of you make is believing that you only need to do aerobics to get that glorious, sexy, defined body. Oh, if it were only true, then anyone who jogs would look great.

But have you ever wondered why most long-distance runners don't have developed bodies, why their muscles aren't firm?

Here we come to the final part of the North Program. There is no better, quicker way to shape, strengthen, and contour the body than with the use of weight training. I don't care how good of an eating plan you follow, and I don't care how many miles you bicycle every day. The best way to get a tight bottom, firm stomach and nice development in the biceps is weight training. Weight training is the easiest body makeover there is. If you want to give yourself a face lift and tummy tuck and narrow hips and thin thighs, then go lift weights. It's less painful and a lot less expensive than surgery.

This is nothing new. But once again, too many of you are plagued by weight-training myths to ever seriously try it. Women think they are going to become over-bloated and muscular (wrong). Men think if they build up too much muscle it will eventually turn to fat (also wrong). Weightlifters who look bloated and fat are not that way because of their weight training. They are that way because of bad eating habits and lack of the proper aerobic exercise.

Only five or six years ago, top athletes were told not to lift weights. Today, the evidence is overwhelming that you need to lift weights at least twice a week. Michael Jordan trains with weights a whopping six days a week—and I don't hear anybody complaining about him being muscle-bound or inflexible. Moreover, the best older athletes—like Nolan Ryan, Jimmy Connors and Martina Navratilova—are also regular weight trainers.

If you're honest with me, you'd tell me that your real problem is you're intimidated about walking into a gym. You see "No Pain, No Gain" posters on the wall. You see all these muscle heads spitting into the water fountain and groaning underneath massive barbells. You see their buddies shouting, "Do just one more! Yeah! Yeah!" You're thinking, My God, if I start doing this, my brain is going to turn to mush and I'm going to act just like these odd people.

No wonder you feel uncomfortable the moment you walk into a gym. You feel lowered self-esteem, you feel far more out of shape compared to the people you see who've been working out there for years. You feel like everyone is staring right at you. And so you do either one of two things: (1) You back up like a crab and disappear forever out the front door or (2) you work out so hard, trying to impress or keep up with everyone around you, that you overdo it and lift far more weight than you're ready for. You end up so sore the next day you can't even get out of bed.

It's doubtful a team of wild horses will ever get you back in a gym.

The Answer

There has to be a reason why, despite the explosion of gyms and health clubs around the country, only 10 percent of the adult population of America has joined them. And barely 10 percent of that group uses their gyms frequently! Why? Could it be that they don't know what true weight training is? Could it finally be time for a rewarding program?

The North Program is going to teach you some surprising new things about how to develop the best muscle. You'll follow a step-by-step program that takes all the intimidation out of weight training and puts the fun back in.

I'm going to teach you that muscle soreness is not a sign of muscle progress. You'll learn the amount of weight is far less important than using the proper form. You'll learn that you need to do this no more than two to three times a week.

You'll tone. Not bulk. You're going to see the muscles develop, not because you're getting huge and muscle-laden, but because your fat layer is shedding.

So here we go, with the only get-lean fitness book you'll ever need. I've outlined our plan of attack, and I know you'll be able to stick with it. The North Program genuinely is the answer—even for those of you who think you are too lazy or don't have the time to do it. As you're about to find out, it's far easier to stay on a lean eating and workout program than it is to stay on any other kind of diet or workout program there is. All you've got to do for me is promise you'll try it. Your answers are only a few pages away.

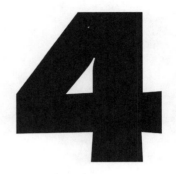

The Diet Myth

Why Your So-Called Diet
Actually Makes You Fatter

How of many of you think that if you take in fewer calories, you'll lose weight more quickly and get a great body? Since thirty-five hundred calories equal a pound, you say, all you have to do is cut out thirty-five hundred calories from your diet and you'll lose another pound. Oh, you poor, misguided souls. If it were really all that simple, then there would not be a flood of diet books at your bookstore. And you would not be reading this one.

The great myth of this industry is that dieting still works. Although every major nutritionist is now saying it doesn't, you are still subjected to television commercials and hotly promoted books about great diet programs and how successful they are. Why? Could it be because there are companies out there that have invested millions of dollars into these programs hoping you'll buy them? They aren't going to suddenly say, "Sorry, guys, we were wrong. We're closing down now and going out of business. Buy that Larry North book, instead."

The fact is, anyone can lose weight. You can do a big crash diet and slim down by ten pounds. There are plenty of programs out there that can give you initial weight loss. But the tragic problem is that it's all destined to come back. Numerous studies now show that people who lose weight through expensive diet programs will gain it all back after one year. Two-thirds will gain their weight back after three years. And the rest will gain it back within five years. What I'm telling you is something you probably don't want to hear. But there is no magical solution to losing weight through a diet. The great danger is that a diet is more likely to put fat on you—exactly the thing you're trying to get rid of.

The Crazy Logic of a Diet

If someone tells me they have lost five pounds in a week, I think, Okay, but what have you lost? Five pounds of water that will come back within days? Five pounds of muscle? Or five pounds of fat?

I admit, if you immediately cut out a bunch of calories from your diet, you will weigh less than you did. But look at what you are taking out. You are not depleting fat but all the water held in your carbohydrate stores. You are losing water weight!

The fact is, you can't permanently lose weight by cutting more and more calories for the rest of your life. I have people who tell me they are so disciplined that they are down to six hundred or seven hundred calories a day. For heaven's sake, that's barely eating. So I say to them, "Well, how's it going?" And they'll inevitably admit, "Well, I lost a lot of weight at first, but now I'm not losing anything."

That's because their bodies have adapted! Once again, allow me to give you a quick science lesson about your own body—a lesson some diet leaders conveniently forget to tell you.

The moment you cut down on calories, your body doesn't know it's supposed to be on a diet. It believes it is starving! Being the amazing machine it is, it starts working to fight starvation. Are you ready for this? The body can double the number of fat storage enzymes and will start trying to hoard more fat than ever before.

Your body also starts to slow down. It's thinking, Hey, I'm famished. I can't use up so much energy. It starts cutting back on its caloric needs. It starts cutting back the speed of its own metabolism. Yes, there's that word again. According to some estimates, if you drop from two thousand calories a day to twelve hundred calories a day, your metabolism decreases by 5 to 10 percent. If you drop down to eight-hundred-calories-a-day diets, your metabolism lowers by 10 to 20 percent.

In other words, if you eat less, you'll need less. All of a sudden, those eight hundred calories a day you're eating will feel, to your own body, like eight thousand calories. Because the metabolism is working at a snail's pace, you can actually start putting on body fat.

The Diet's Second Sucker Punch

Wait, I'm not yet finished with this horror story. There's no question that diets will make your body, now desperately looking for nutrients, deplete its carbohydrate cells (which includes all your water weight). But that's not much of a help. You want to get rid of fat, not carbohydrates. But disastrously, after the carbohydrates are gone, your body still doesn't go into its fat stores. It heads toward its own stores of muscle tissue to look for protein.

In other words, your diet isn't taking off fat. The more you diet, the more you are cutting into your own valuable muscle. Indeed, up to 50 percent of the weight you lose can come from muscle. A diet is like a double whammy—for as you already know, less muscle will slow down the metabolism even more.

Wait! There's more bad news. I mean really bad.

With your new slower metabolism rate, you've got a greater chance than ever before to regain all your weight back. The minute you eat something again, two things will happen:

1. Your depleted carbohydrate cells, desperate to soak up any fluid they can, will act like sponges, and you'll get a huge amount of fluid retention—meaning your water weight soars back up; and

2. Your slowed metabolic rate won't be able to speed up in time to burn off the new food you have just put in, which means the food will go right to your fat cells! Your fat cells expand as your muscle cells simultaneously shrink. With more fat in your

body than muscle, your body doesn't need as much energy to keep itself going, which means the metabolism rate slows down even more!

Holy moly, tell me right now you are still interested in dieting. If you are, keep reading, because I have got even worse news.

Knockout!

When your diet fails and you start putting on the poundage in the form of fat, you now have more fat to lose in your next diet. When you blow that diet and gain weight again, you're putting on even more fat than before. Moreover, each time you go on a diet (and reports say the average dieter goes on 2.3 diets per year), it takes longer for your body to lose the weight and faster to regain it.

You're in a vicious cycle. I have seen women who have been on so many low-calorie diets that they have an abnormally high fat-muscle ratio. They can actually gain weight if they starve. Such a yo-yo pattern of dieting—losing and regaining, losing and regaining—was found, in one study, to have significantly increased the risk of heart disease.

Plus, the places where you regain weight is frustrating. Fat, it has been said, is like a river. It's going to flow right to that part of the body that has the least resistance. So for men, it will go to the middle, creating those hated pot bellies. For women, it will go to the buttocks and thighs—exactly what got you started dieting in the first place. Just because you take in less calories does not mean you're going to reshape those problem areas.

But You Say You Have Willpower?

I know, despite everything I've said, that there are still some of you die-hard dieters who are saying, "Sorry, Larry, I've got the ability to stay with a low-calorie diet. I'm not going to yo-yo. I'm going to stay this weight for the rest of my life." No, you're not. There is no study that has found someone who's able to permanently beat back obesity with a low-calorie diet. In fact, you have probably dieted so much that you have taught your body to ignore its natural biological signals that tell you when you're hungry and when you're full. Inevitably, you're going to eat something. And when you do, your body doesn't know when to stop eating. You binge.

I would like to know why people go to such great lengths to be unhappy. When you diet, you cannot help but think and dream about food. You're likely to suffer wide mood swings. You wonder why you can't lose five more pounds. You often become depressed, anxious and irritable.

And then what do you do? You turn to food as your emotional salve. The more you obsess about not eating, the more you are really thinking about food—so when you give yourself the chance to put food in your body, you blow it.

But, you say, at least I only ate one big meal. That's wrong, too. As I'll later explain, it's a lot worse for you to eat one huge meal than several small ones spaced throughout a day.

The North Body Shop

I want you, from now on, to think of your body as an engine. The more pure fuel you put in (and the key word is "pure"), the more the fire will heat up and the hotter the engine will burn. If you put in less pure fuel, the engine slows.

I also want you to think of your fat cells as very smart, very ingenious clogs in that engine. No matter what service station you've been to before, the fat cells have figured out how to beat you.

Now it's time to get to the North Body Shop. We are going to turn your body into a fuel-efficient engine, where you put plenty of the right kind of calories into your body. You're going to send those calories straight to your engine and not into your fat cells.

You have paid a terrible price for years of nutritional misinformation. You still don't know what to eat and when to eat it. But if you follow the plan I'm going to give you later in this book, if you eat the kinds of foods you need to stoke up your engine, then you're going to find yourself building muscle and increasing your metabolism.

You can achieve results permanently without completely destroying your life. It isn't going to take a supreme effort. It won't require you to suffer the pangs of hunger or the yo-yos of dieting.

It's time to get started.

Getting Started

The First Steps
to Reshaping Your Body

Some of you haven't worked out in years—and here I am, asking you to lift weights. Some of you have been practicing the one-meal-a-day diet—and here I am, asking you to eat five or six meals a day. I'm also telling you this is your program for life! Feeling down yet? Think it's impossible? Aren't you just a tiny bit upset that I'm not promising you the perfect look in only six weeks? Listen, if you are still thinking in that old negative fashion, then put my book aside, go buy one of those "Fabulous Secret Diet Plan for Your Life" books, and when you realize that you're being misled again, come on back to me.

Back so soon?

All right, as I was saying, if you cannot, at this moment, walk out the door and down to your corner mailbox without huffing and puffing, then welcome. You're just the person I want to see. If you believe you're in reasonably good shape but don't know why you can't get over that hump to develop a sensational body, then welcome. I want to see you, too.

First, though, I want everyone to relax. I'm not going to ask you to do anything superhuman. Don't feel like you ought to do a month or two of push-ups before you try the North Program. I know that, for now, none of this is going to feel easy, but this program really does allow you to use the talents you have regardless of how listless or out of shape you think you are.

Okay, now we're moving. In truth, the first mistake almost everyone makes when starting a program is that they have no plan. That's like building a house without blueprints, or trying to build it from the tenth floor down. Now that you know where we're heading, here's the next thing I want you to do:

Get on a good pair of walking or running shoes, take a watch with you and walk out the door at a comfortable pace. Put on headphones if you want and listen to music. Walk for thirty minutes. If you feel terribly overweight and out of shape, then walk five minutes out your door and five minutes back. Congratulations. The fat-burning process, in that walk, has been accelerated. It's breaking the ice. It's like going to the driving range to get the golf swing ready.

Your First Excuse

Now, you're two days into the program, you've leafed through the book, and you're thinking about giving the North Program a shot. So you're saying, "Hmm, maybe I should go get all those stress tests and heart tests."

I know that a lot of fitness books, tend to scare you by suggesting you see a doctor before you begin the program—just to make sure you won't drop over dead going through it. Look, I'm not asking you to start an Olympic training program here. I'm not going to ask for huge exertion. I certainly hope that you are getting an annual physical with a doctor, especially if you are over forty. And if you feel you might have a problem—heart condition, diabetes, osteoporosis, back problem, bad knees—then by all means, go see a doctor before starting this program. But for those of you who know you can walk for thirty minutes, who know you can go do a light weight routine—then the idea that you have to wait until you see a doctor is only an excuse.

Besides, if you're forty years old, out of shape and you eat like the typical baby boomer, what the heck do you think a doctor is going to tell you? He's going to tell you to get on an exercise program.

Furthermore, forget about all those tests that you can get in health clubs. You don't need a scientific fat test. You don't need a pulse-rate test on a treadmill.

Here's what you need to do. It's the Larry North Fat Test, free of charge. Pull up your shirt and stare at your stomach. Using your thumb and forefinger, pinch a spot beneath your lowest rib and a couple of inches from your side. If the gap between your thumb and forefinger is greater than an inch, you are overweight.

Here's a better test. Take your clothes off and look at yourself in the mirror. Are you happy with that? No? Then let's get after it.

Your Second Mission

Now that you know you have body fat, you need to figure out how it got there. Most of you, I've discovered, have utterly no idea what you eat or what kind of exercising you do. Merely by starting a couple of journals, your awareness will not only soar, but you will already find yourself changing some bad habits.

1. Start an exercise journal. Record the times you work out and what you do. When you keep a written record of your workout sessions, it will make a big difference in your long-term success. You'll start enjoying the pattern of your workouts more; you'll hate it when you break the regularity. You'll see your workouts like a bank account deposit. Each deposit might not mean much—but taken together over a year, the deposit can add up to huge savings.

2. Start a food journal. Write down what you eat through an entire day. Studies show that by having to write down what you eat, you automatically eat better foods. Plus, as you learn more about eating, you will use this journal to see exactly which foods you're relying on that need to be replaced—such as what fatty foods you want when you give in to a craving. You might discover that you already eat a nutritionally balanced

meal except for some high-fat meals at the end of the day. Your journals need not be permanent—keep them for the first six to twelve weeks of the program. In other words, keep them long enough so you'll know what you need to work on.

Your Third Mission

This is going to seem odd. But I want you to go visit a gym or a health club. Don't put on workout clothes, and make sure there's not a salesman or instructor hanging over you. Just sit back and watch the action.

Although I'm going to show you later how to set up a simple, functional weight area in your own home (if that's what you prefer), I always recommend that you still go to a health club periodically to work on weight machines that you might not have. Moreover, I want you to notice something. Besides some personal trainers and a few long-time veterans, you'll see that most everyone else there is struggling just like you. Walk around. You'll notice that people don't care whether someone is lifting a five-pound dumbbell or a one-hundred-pound one.

What still astonishes me, in every gym I've been to, is the way strangers will encourage others, no matter what their level of fitness. A weight room can seem like the last friendly community, sort of a small town. Someone will help you work on your form; someone else will help you change a weight. You won't understand this until you experience it. But please—don't let the muscle magazines and the bodybuilding physiques intimidate you. There's more than enough room for you.

Fourth Mission

Go buy some workout clothes you feel you look nice in. I'm not telling you to buy the most expensive designer outfit. But get something to wear so you don't feel self conscious about your body. The baggier the better, if that's what you want. Sorry to use a cliché, but if you look good, you feel good. And that will make you a lot more comfortable when we get to the weight room.

Those Frightening Scales

The next thing I want you to do is to forget about weighing yourself. That's right. Put your bathroom scales up in your closet. Spending your days jumping on and off scales can make you totally neu-rotic—and if there is one thing you need to work on, it's to make your North Program fun, not anxiety-ridden.

If you jump on a scale one morning and you're three pounds heavier than usual, you might spend the rest of the day in a terrible mood. Or, if you wake up and find you're two pounds less than usual, you might be so thrilled you'll allow yourself a fattening fast-food breakfast sandwich.

The problem with scales is that they tend to gauge your water weight, which is always variable. I'm not concerned with how much you weigh. I'm concerned with your body fat. You lose fat in ounces. Conventional scales don't measure ounces; they measure pounds. They can't distinguish water weight from fat weight. Moreover, it is quite possible that as you progress in this program, you will weigh more on a scale even while you lose body fat, because lean muscle tissue weighs more than fat. (And don't forget that you can lose weight and still gain body fat.)

So, if you focus on scales, you won't be focusing on your whole body—its proportion and shape. And that's what I'm concerned with—whether you're getting tighter around the waist and fuller in the chest. Forget all those silly charts that say if you're a certain height, then you should be a certain weight. You can weigh the same as you did twenty years ago, but your waistline might be five inches wider.

The Inevitable Silly Weight Question

There's another thing that always bothers me. It's that question a lot of personal trainers always ask you when you get started in a program: "How much weight do you want to lose?"

Don't worry about it. With the North Program, the weight loss will come—sometimes fast, sometimes slow. I know a lot of you immediately want to know, "Larry, when can I expect to go from 130 pounds to 110 pounds?" And I say that if your program depends on losing exactly a certain amount of weight, then you are going to fail. You'll always be disappointed, and you'll be more likely to give up. Everybody has a different genetic makeup, which makes it impossible to uniformly say how much you're going to lose.

Stay patient. Our fat didn't show up on our bodies overnight, nor will it come off overnight—regardless of what a thousand fitness hucksters have told you. I want you to learn to enjoy the long, great process of shaping your body. You don't have to give yourself a goal to lose ten pounds in a month. You know what your goal is: to look good, to lose body fat, to get rid of that bulge, to feel better and to fit into clothes that make you feel attractive.

A program that can permanently keep excess body fat off you is a program that asks for small changes. If you go any faster trying to lose weight, you'll find yourself losing water weight or precious muscle rather than body fat. What I want to tell you, as you begin this journey, is to keep focused on your body. If you knew the weight issue would take care of itself as long as you kept getting fit and eating right, then wouldn't that be a lot easier?

What? Did You Say Cheat Already?

As I said before, I'm not going to hide anything from you. The price of this program—the price of staying lean—is eternal vigilance. But for those of you still thinking the North Program is going to be way too strict, let me say four shocking words:

It's okay to cheat. I know there is going to come a time when you won't feel like you're watching yourself like a guard dog. I know you are going to cheat. Anyone who is in this business and says you can stick 100 percent to a program is a fool. Those are people who literally don't know what the real world is like. It is impossible to eat perfectly all the time. And you are not always going to get in your workouts.

When most people start a program, they feel they fail whenever they stray—and they think they need to start all over again. But remember: the North Program is not pass or fail. *You don't fail at this program, you just get better at it.* Getting the North Body takes as long as it has to take—but it is going to work.

I don't want any of you reading this book to think that you are a failure if you are not following the strictest aspects of this program. Just the fact that you will know when you are "cheating" is, at the start, a big plus. It indicates that you have learned to distinguish good eating from bad. You know how to choose.

You, the reader of this book, get to dictate how much you eat, how many calories you take in, how many desserts you avoid. And if you go and have a blowout, high-fat dinner on Sunday night? It's not the end of the world. On Monday morning you just get back on the program again.

Still Don't Want to Start?

Come on, you can tell me. Are you really hesitant to get going? Have you been talking to someone who is telling you that all the exercise in the world won't guarantee you an extra day of life? Someone who's saying that eating properly only means you'll eat bland, boring foods? Are you out of your mind?

Do I need to remind you that being overweight is associated with a greater risk of high blood pressure? By managing your weight, you might be able to prevent one of the most prevalent diseases (hypertension) in our nation today.

Do you need to be told again that too much fat in your body places a strain on the heart, causing increased cholesterol in your blood and raising your chance for heart disease? That fat in your body leads to arthritis, gall bladder disease, some forms of diabetes, and loads of psychological stress that comes from feeling overweight and unattractive? That women with high body fat have a greater risk for breast cancer? That men with pot bellies are more likely to have heart attacks?

Let me remind you what is going to happen to you if you do not start this program. To repeat an old Jack La Lanne phrase about working out, "If you don't use it, you're going to lose it." Your body will wear out, plain and simple, like an old machine—not worn out from use, but worn out from rust. For you not to take responsibility for a fitness plan is to invite personal disaster. The more you work out, the more your long-dormant muscle tissue will grow, rejuvenating itself. New muscle tissue will grow. You'll regain elasticity and strength. You will live better than you've ever lived before.

The Gary Hotchkiss Story

If you really think you're not capable of doing this program, even after everything I've told you, then I want you to meet Gary Hotchkiss, an accountant who owns his own successful firm and lectures on financial topics around the country. For two years, in the privacy of his home, he listened to my radio show, taking in all the information I put out regarding proper nutrition and exercise. He debated with himself whether this was for him.

Finally, he got the courage to make an appointment for a consultation with me at my gym in Dallas.

I could not believe what I was seeing. Gary Hotchkiss was incredibly overweight—445 pounds! He barely fit through the door! I wondered what he felt like walking through my gym, past lots of people diligently working out, and then sitting precariously down on a chair to say to me, "Larry, what can I do?"

At that point, I had worked with hundreds of people. I had given them specific eating and weight-training plans that tremendously changed their bodies. For a moment, looking at Gary, I thought,

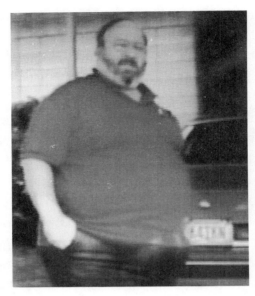

"Well, here's the ultimate test case to see if the North Program really works. If he can succeed, absolutely anyone can succeed."

Gary already had tried the usual fasting and low-calorie diets. In one diet, he lost fifty pounds in only two months—and, of course, gained it all back a few months later. Other instructors had told him not to exercise, even mildly, because they were afraid he'd get hurt. I said, "Gary, nothing is going to work as quickly as an exercise and eating program. We're going to destroy that body fat."

At his first workout, he walked for five minutes on a treadmill at the lowest speed possible. He was so out of breath that he could barely take another step. He couldn't do any weight machines because he couldn't fit in them!

To almost everyone in the gym, Gary's situation seemed hopeless. But here was the key. He wanted to change. Gary did what you are going to have to do—he made a conscious decision that he was not going to look bad again.

He started eating small, low-fat meals six times a day. He didn't starve himself. But he did what it took to make sure he kept the fat out of his diet. He learned to special order in restaurants, just as you will learn to do. He learned to pre-prepare healthy nonfat meals, just as you will.

He began a small weight program and soon was carrying a set of dumbbells with him on the road when he regularly traveled for business. Often when he was out of town, he'd look up a gym in the Yellow Pages and go work out there. He also began a walking program, nothing more and nothing less. He realized he could walk anywhere in the country, that he never had to worry about missing a workout. Within eight weeks, he was walking forty-five minutes a day. Soon after that, he was walking at a sixty-minute pace so fast that his own twenty-year-old daughter couldn't keep up with him.

Gary Hotchkiss's body changed—permanently. In his first seven months on the program, he lost 190 pounds.

Now, here's the great news. Gary Hotchkiss (who has lost thirty-four inches off his waist and is down to 218 pounds) did nothing more than what I'm going to show you in the rest of this book. He didn't radically change his life. He just made some alterations in his eating habits, took an hour to get in his workouts—and he demolished his body fat.

This is not one of those cheap before-and-after stories you read about in magazine ads. This is the real thing. No diet, no three-a-day workouts in the weight room, no medically supervised treatment. It was just the North Program.

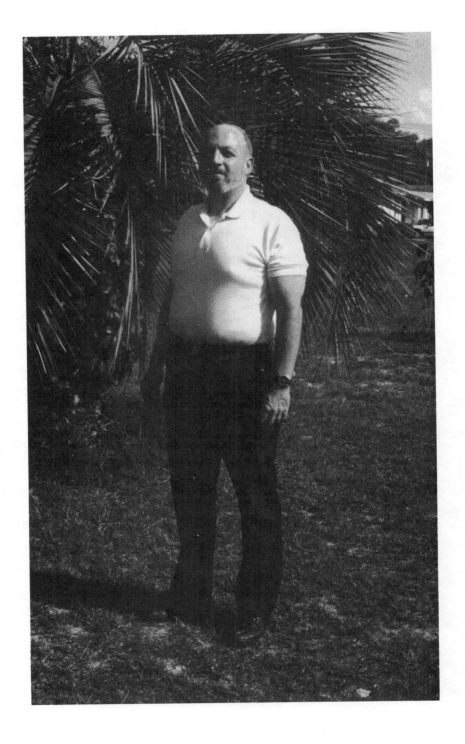

Pure Fuel for Your Engine

Taking the Mystery out of
Nutrition and Moving
into the Larry North Program

f you've done any reading about nutrition at all, then I'm sure you're confused. One plan tells you to eat only twenty grams of fat per day. Another program tells you to make sure 30 percent of your diet is fat. Wait, here's a program saying it should be 20 percent fat. And here's one saying to forget fat grams, but to count calories. Eat eighteen hundred calories a day. No, says someone else, make that twelve hundred calories a day.

Yikes. Nutrition sounds like a guessing game. It also sounds like a lot of hogwash, especially when you are inundated with ads from breakfast cereals that claim they are "vitamin enriched" when in fact they are 52 percent sugar. Or what about all these products that claim they are "low fat" when in fact they are a half-gram lower in fat than they used to be.

Please, let me make this a no-brainer for you. It's not that I don't think nutrition is important—what you eat is going to determine whether you're successful in the North Program—but you don't need these complicated five-hundred-page nutrition books to figure it all out.

First, stop counting calories and fat grams. That's right. Once again, I'm saying something that sounds like sacrilege in the health industry. But it's time to get rid of this crazy idea of nutrition as math. All of you who are out there worrying whether you ate too many calories or fat grams yesterday, forget it. Calorie and fat gram counting is not practical. It requires that you know how many calories are in every single morsel of food you eat. Moreover, the effect of caloric intake depends on so many variables—the amount of muscle you already have, your ability to digest food, your present metabolic rate. And unless you are prepared to read an encyclopedia—or get a muscle biopsy and blood and body fat testing every other week—then you need something more practical and effective.

The Alternative

Though I carefully watch what I eat, I don't count calories or fat grams. I mainly avoid fat and sugar. I avoid them like big mean dogs in the street.

The issue is not cutting calories. It's keeping as much fat as possible out of your diet. And if you know how to pick the right amount of foods from the right food groups—and no, I'm not talking about the antiquated "four basic food groups"—then you are going to be successful. Plain and simple.

In my book, there's simply two things you need to know about nutrition: (1) the kinds of right foods you should eat, and (2) the kinds of fatty foods to avoid.

The North Body Foods

To get the North Body, you must eat:

1. *Complex Carbohydrates.* That includes brown rice, yams, grits, white potatoes, sweet potatoes, oatmeal, oat bran, corn, whole-grain breads, whole-grain pastas, shredded wheat and dried legumes such as pinto beans, black-eyed peas, lima beans and black beans, white, navy and kidney beans.

2. *Proteins.* That includes cuts of turkey breast, white chicken, white fishes, egg whites and only the very leanest cuts of red meat.

3. *Fibrous Vegetables.* That includes broccoli, cauliflower, carrots, green and red peppers, asparagus, celery, spinach,

lettuces, green peas, egg plant, green beans, squash, cabbage, mushrooms, radishes, Brussels sprouts, onions, zucchini, cucumbers, etc.

If your eating program consists of one serving of a lean protein, one complex carbohydrate and one fibrous vegetable at each meal (and you can occasionally throw in a piece of fruit), you'll get lean so fast your head will spin. And that, ladies and gentlemen, is all you need to know. I'm quite serious.

Your First Fears

I always love the look on people's faces when they first see such a list. They scream, "This is it? That's what Larry North wants me to eat for the rest of my life?"

Take a deep breath and relax. All I'm asking you to do, right now, is keep reading—not to nosedive into some new kind of eating program. We're just taking tiny steps at the moment—but by the end of this book, I bet you're going to want to eat perfectly.

Besides, if you look over that food list again, you're going to find that you probably don't eat drastically differently. Most experts, in stressing the importance of proper food, fail to emphasize how little needs to be taken out of the diet to produce tangible results over a long period of time. In the North Program you are going to find you will eat most of the same foods you've eaten before, only you are going to have them prepared differently.

A Very Simple Nutrition Lesson

I want you to understand why you need a balance of carbohydrates, protein and fat, because I believe if you genuinely understand what various foods do to you, then you'll want to follow the program more carefully. Let's review a few relevant terms:

Complex Carbohydrates (also known as "starchy carbs" or "starches" or "carbs") comprise the basic energy for your body.

They are broken down, after entering the body, into glucose, which is the stuff burned as fuel inside every cell. Remember the image of our bodies as engines, needing the purest of fuels? Carbs are the most efficiently burned fuel you can put into your body. They build up and increase your metabolism. Because you have limited capacity to store carbs, almost all the carbs you eat are burned within a few hours (unless, of course, you seriously overeat).

Protein is also critical for your body. It repairs injured muscle fibers, and provides additional amino acids to build more muscle. It's necessary to help control the conversion of carbohydrates into glucose. Protein also provides the right kind of energy to build your muscles. Protein becomes important as your weight training begins because it is necessary to replenish your muscles that get exercised.

Fibrous Vegetables: You have got to have fibrous veggies in your diet because that is where most of your nutrition really lies—the vitamins and the enzymes. Fiber-rich foods also require more energy to digest, which increases the rate at which calories are burned. And because they are digested more slowly, they help you to feel full more quickly.

Your body requires some fat; these are called "the essential fatty acids." But you do not have to eat fatty foods to get those fatty acids. Most of the food groups I've already mentioned contain some amount of fat. *You don't need to add anything in your eating to get the proper fat in.*

Indeed, with every extra pound of fat you take in, you're adding a lot of extra blood vessels in your body—miles of them. These blood vessels drain away the very blood you need to work through your other body organs. That means there is more of a strain on your heart. That's why overweight people tend to die earlier and easier than people who stay in shape.

Fat Gram Hell

Aha, I see your busy mind at work. All those misconceptions you've developed over the years still haven't left you completely. You're saying, "Uh, Larry, don't I need to cut all foods besides fat to lose weight? Don't I need to cut down on my proteins and carbs, and vegetables, too? Is cutting back fat enough? Don't I need to cut calories all the way around?"

Oh, yes, the old all-calories-are-the-same myth.

Here's the truth: Not all calories are created equal. Just this once I'm going to do some calorie counting for you, but only to prove a point. When you eat a gram of fat, you're taking in nine calories! That's more than twice as many calories that come from a gram of carbohydrate or a gram of protein.

If you eat only two thousand calories a day, but you get it all from high-fat food like potato chips and steak, then you are in serious trouble. "Fat calories" (calories that come from fatty food) will go straight to your fat cells. Some studies say that 97 percent of all fat calories you take in will be converted into body fat. In other words, if you eat one hundred calories of fat above the proper amount your body needs, your body will burn only three of them. Three calories!

And never forget, it's a lot easier to overeat fat than overeat other foods. Once you get started on a good piece of high-fat food—like a bowl of ice cream—you will discover that you just put down hundreds of calories.

The Moment of Truth

So now we come to the grand revelation. If you get your calories from carbs and proteins, then those calories get used far more quickly. I mean, gosh, this is so simple. In the North Program, you get to eat a lot more food—you get to take in a lot more calories— because you are eating food that gets burned up by your fuel-efficient engine. All you need to know is what foods you should reduce or avoid. We are going to remove fat, sugar and processed foods. And then you replace them with the right type of foods you should eat—at every meal, you have a protein, some type of complex carb, and some sort of fibrous vegetable. Bang. Just as I said: a no-brainer.

I'm not saying you can't have fatty foods when you have a craving for them. It just means you are going to try to reduce your consumption of these foods to a minimum. Gloriously, if you do that, you will not need to burden yourself with calorie counting to know you are below 10 percent of your caloric intake in fat.

Then What Do I Eliminate?

Later in another chapter, I'm going to be more specific about which fat-laden foods you need to get rid of, and what foods you can use as substitutes, and ways to make certain foods low fat. But for now, there are some general categories you need to learn.

1. *Oils.* Try to keep oil to a bare minimum. That includes salad dressings, vegetable cooking oils, butter and margarine. A single tablespoon of that oil contains 120 calories of fat—a tablespoon! If you must use oil, look for monosaturated and polyunsaturated oils. Don't use saturated oils.

2. *Sugar.* Obviously, you want to get rid of simple sugars, like candies and fruit juices, because they can go straight into your bloodstream and to your fat cells without ever being broken down by the body. Try to take out all forms of sugars, which includes dextrose, glucose, suchrose, honey, molasses, pure cane sugar, white sugar or refined sugar.

3. *Processed foods.* Usually, that means anything that comes in a box or in a can, such as cold cuts, crackers, chips, cookies, packaged macaroni and cheese, breads, pastas, white flour products and most boxes of cereal. Almost-processed foods have loads of added oil or sugar. Processed foods take vitamins and fibers and minerals and replace them with preservatives, artificial flavorings and other additives. Many processed

foods are, indeed, good sources of starchy carbs, but by the time they are mixed, mashed, and boxed, those foods become extremely calorically dense. You'll only hurt your program if you rely completely on processed carbohydrates including pastas and bread. (Canned tuna in water, white meat chicken, and veggies without fat or sugar are all okay.)

4. *Dairy.* You'll want to make your dairy products a condiment, not a staple. It is virtually impossible to lose weight while consuming an array of cheeses and milk. Whole milk contains 49.2 percent fat calories. Two percent milk means you're getting 2 percent less fat than whole milk, but that's still 34.9 percent fat calories.

5. *Specific high-fat natural foods.* Such plant foods as avocados, olives, nuts and seeds are all loaded with fat. The minute you eliminate those foods, the better off you'll be.

How Boring Is This?

People always ask me if I ever get tired of eating the same thing. No. People who eat junk always eat the same junk. I say, "Look, you're using the very same foods I am. They're just prepared differently." Instead of a chicken fried steak with mashed potatoes, gravy and broccoli casserole, I go for a grilled, non-oiled chicken with a baked potato and broccoli. The truth is that there has never been a better time to order great-tasting low-fat meals from restaurants and learn how to cook the low-fat way.

Imagine this: you have one shot glass full of cooking oil, another shot glass full of melted butter, you have a shot glass full of mayonnaise, and you have a shot glass full of sugar. All the North Program does is take those shot glasses out of your diet. You're still going to get some oil and sugar in your diet—you can't help it.

But drink a shot glass of oil and tell me how good that tastes. Now tell me how boring this program is.

And Who Said You Had to Eat Three Square Meals a Day?

I also want you once again to turn traditional diet thinking on its head. The only way you can get lean is to eat more meals a day than you normally do. In fact, eat twice as many.

The idea that our meals should consist of three long meals—breakfast, lunch and dinner—is as outdated as the idea that losing weight merely requires losing calories. It's outdated for two reasons:

1. *Eating Less Leads to Overeating.* If you eat only three meals per day—and I know a lot of people who try to eat just two—then you're keeping food from your body for up to six hours at a time. Your body will be so famished that by the time you take in food again, you will overeat. Let's say you miss meals through the day. By the evening, you are going to blow it out. It's a physical impossibility not to.

   Let's say you're trying to get lean and you have a cup of coffee and toast for breakfast. Then you eat a salad and yogurt for lunch. Then you go from 1:00 p.m. to 7:00 p.m. without eating. When you walk into the house, exhausted and hungry, what do you think you're going to want to eat? Certainly not a grilled chicken breast with steamed broccoli and brown rice. You are craving fat and sugar. This is a physical need—not just a psychological one. Your body is shutting down and requires energy—and sugar is one of the quickest ways to get a quick, energetic high.

   If you haven't given yourself nutrients throughout the day, you are going to crave something to keep your energy up, and that's naturally something high in fat. You also want something that is instantly satisfying, that fills you up quickly. And that can also mean fat. The reason you always feel stuffed from a meal is not because you ate too much. It's because you've eaten large amounts of fat.

2. *Eating Less Increases Your Ability to Store Fat.* There are many of you who have told me that you have discipline. "Look, Larry," you say, "I can hold myself to two meals a day, maybe even one big meal a day. I'm tough." You're thinking that if you eat one big meal, perhaps at midday, then your body will easily work through that and then work on your extra fat for the rest of the day.

That's just not the way your body works. A big meal swamps your body's digestive system. The extra food that it cannot digest or process will head straight to the fat cells. For example, you might consume one thousand calories in one sitting. But your body might be able to handle only six hundred calories at a time. That additional four hundred would have to be stored as fat.

Here you are faced with the vicious cycle. Craving food after being neglected for many hours, your body sends signals asking you to overindulge. Once you overindulge, your body is overwhelmed and sends the food to fat. The way to guard against new fat cells is to avoid large intakes of food at one time.

I don't want you to get confused about this, so let me say one more thing. Even if you eat too much of the *right* foods in one sitting, your overloaded body will turn it to fat. Your body can only handle so much protein and carbohydrates at a time, no matter how good they are for you.

The Answer

That's why smaller, frequent meals are critically important, all of them spaced out throughout the day. I'm not saying to eat more food. I want you to eat more frequently.

My plan for you is to build up to five to six smaller meals a day. If you do, you'll have more energy because your blood sugar level remains stable. Because you're regularly eating, you won't ever feel like you're starving enough to lose control when you sit down for a meal. And breaking up meals allows your body to work best at absorbing the necessary nutrients. The body can better utilize such things as protein from smaller amounts of food every two or three hours during the day.

Most importantly, if you do this meal plan, you speed up your all-important metabolism. You're sending in pure amounts of fuel into your engine at regular intervals. Just like putting too much wood on a fire can snuff it out, putting too much food into your body can slow down the engine. Don't forget the earlier lesson: the longer you wait between meals, then the slower your metabolism becomes. And also remember that when you eat a huge meal, you become more sedentary. After such a meal, a great amount of blood is drawn to the digestive tract to try to absorb the food. That means less blood goes to the brain or to the muscles. And that ultimately means you have less energy. You turn into one of those post-meal zombies.

The worst sin you can commit on the eating program is miss meals. It is an absolute no-no. Going long stretches of time without eating will sabotage your program. That is why I will tell you that missing a meal is as big of a "cheat" as eating a high fat meal.

What To Do Right Now

Try something for me. Without changing the makeup of the food you presently eat, just start spreading that food into smaller, more frequent meals. If you take the same food you eat in three meals, and space it out through five or six meals, you won't get as chubby. You will actually start to get leaner—and that's without yet eating the right foods.

You don't believe me? There was a study done in which two groups of rats were given the same amount of food. One group got it in one meal, and the other group got it in five meals. The five-meal group actually lost fat and increased muscle. Just imagine what's going to happen to your body when you choose the right kinds of foods and schedule them to be eaten throughout the day. If there's ever a "secret" to the North Program, this is it.

But How Do I Do It?

Good question. How in the world do you eat five or six meals per day, which means eating every three hours? You're probably thinking that you'll end up overeating far more than you do now. You're saying, "There's no way I can do that many meals. I barely have time for three meals a day."

I've heard these excuses a thousand times. Can't do it. Too busy. Too many kids to take care of. Blah, blah. Let me take out my violin.

The fact is, if you include your little snacks, you probably eat five or six times a day already. I'll bet my savings on it. Whether it's a bag of chips, a candy bar, a yogurt, you're still eating. Let me give you a typical baby boomer eating plan:

Morning: Nothing. He skips breakfast altogether because he's hustling to work.

Midmorning: Coffee and a bran muffin. He thinks a bran muffin is good because it has bran, when the fact is it has ten to fifteen grams of fat. That's enormous.

Lunch: A standard lunch. It could be anything from a cheeseburger to a club sandwich to Mexican food to a Lean Cuisine which he thinks is so good for him.

Midday: A candy bar or pack of potato chips or piece of fruit. Maybe, if it's been a bad day, he'll have all three.

Dinner: A traditional meal of a meat, vegetables, salad, a dessert, wine and/or beer.

Late-night snack: Ice cream or a bowl of cereal.

That, my friends, is a five-meal day. Doesn't sound that bad, right?

Unfortunately, this person, if he eats like that 365 days a year, is going to pile up fat for the next ten years. If I could take this person's day, and knock out some of the fats, and add a nonfat morning meal, his body would change.

If he was following my plan, he'd want to eat five or six times a day, because (1) he wouldn't be eating much fat (which makes a person feel more satiated than carbs or proteins), and (2) his metabolism would be working faster. That means he'd burn through his food quicker and get hungry faster, ready for that next meal in three hours. And instead of his emotional and physical stamina plummeting with a diet, he would feel terrific.

So, from now on, there will be no calorie counting, no diets, no Fit for Life, no Diet Center. It's time to learn the best eating plan on the face of this earth.

The Larry North Meal Plan:
You've Been Taught How to Diet. Now Learn How to Eat

Just to show you what a no-brainer program this is, let me take you through a day of eating—a perfect five-meal day for me.

8:00 a.m.: I ate breakfast at a restaurant, ordering a bowl of oatmeal, two pieces of dry toast and five egg whites (all the fat of an egg is in the yellowish yolk, and the white has pure protein, but no fat.)

11:00 a.m.: I had a steamed chicken breast, a plain baked potato and steamed broccoli.

2:00 p.m.: I ate a grilled chicken breast (cooked without oil), steamed cabbage, a salad with nonfat lemon dressing, and green beans.

5:00 p.m.: After a workout, I stopped at a grocery store and bought five hard-boiled eggs, rice cakes, a package of baby carrots, a bottle of purified water, and two pieces of sliced honeydew melon—a meal, incidentally, which cost less than five dollars.

8:30 p.m.: At home, I had a cup of rice, a broiled chicken breast and spinach.

You could possibly come up with meals that might have the same amount of calories as the meals I ate—like a ground beef patty and some slices of nonfat white bread. But will that food help you become lean? Is it the right fuel for your engine? Of course not. If you noticed, I was not eating a lot.

The Need for Balance

Each meal has to be balanced. Don't underestimate the importance of this. At every meal you must have a serving of protein, a serving of a complex carbohydrate, and a fibrous vegetable.

I see a lot of people sabotage their program by overdosing on carbs like pastas and breads. If you eat too many carbs and too little protein at a meal, you'll overstuff your body and you won't get lean. On the other hand, some people eat a lot of carbs in the first or second meals, but then cut back on carbs through the rest of the day—which can make them end up feeling very listless and hungry, and in danger of overeating at the next meal. Some people just don't eat enough carbs, which makes their bodies crave sweets. The key is to evenly spread out your foods.

A balanced meal plan also means to space the meals out evenly through the day. Don't eat three quick meals in the morning and then two in the evening. Do your best to eat every three hours.

Finally, a balanced meal plan means the size of each meal has to be balanced. You can't eat one large meal to start off the day and make your next meal smaller. They all need to be approximately the same size.

There's always a controversy about some food groups—such as proteins. Some nutritionists will tell you to eat more protein; some will say less. But they all agree that if you're highly athletic, you need more protein. They also say you must space your protein out in smaller meals throughout the day.

Your Plan

What I'm going to give you is a six-week plan to learn to eat perfectly. It is going to start slowly and eventually get tougher.

The only way you'll know this can work is to try it. So don't deviate from the program for the next six weeks. By the sixth week, you'll be on the ideal meal plan. I want you to know what it's like, at that six-week point, to get your body's metabolism fired to its prime level. I'm not going to expect you to eat that way all the time. If you want to be less severe after that first six weeks, that's fine. Add a few items back in. But don't lose the basic goal of the program. If you need to snack between meals during this six weeks, then eat plain rice cakes, carrots and celery sticks.

Don't expect yourself to be 100 percent successful as you get into this. It takes a while to change bad eating habits. Taking it slow is only going to help you. And remember, if during this period you miss a meal, it doesn't mean you have blown your program for the day. Just pick right back up where you left off.

Week One

In the first week, I want you to cut back on your sugary drinks like alcohol, soft drinks and fruit juice (which is basically sugar water once the fruit fiber has been removed). Try to drink water as a substitute. That's it. If you need to, write down those three items on a sheet of paper and carry it with you everywhere you go. Don't think about cutting anything else out.

The only other thing I want you to do is to be able to identify what has fat in it—all of the oils, salad dressings and fried foods. Be aware of what you're eating. Recognize that you're massively adding to the fat of a slice of bread just by spreading a thin layer of butter across it.

Now try to increase your meal frequency. Whatever you can get in for the day is great. Remember, nothing in the first week should feel difficult. All you want to do is attempt to eat a little more healthily. Here's a sample day's eating program:

Meal One (or breakfast): Cereal with skim milk, two whole eggs with two additional egg whites, two slices of toast with jam.

Meal Two (or lunch): A turkey sandwich with mustard (never mayonnaise), a bowl of rice and a salad with lemon or vinegar dressing.

Snack: A piece of fruit.

Meal Four (or dinner): A meat such as white fish, a potato, corn and a salad with lemon or vinegar dressing.

Late-night Snack: A bowl of oatmeal.

In Week One, you can have three cheat meals. They can be anything you want. Don't overdo it and create a smorgasbord for yourself. Eat only a regular-sized cheat meal.

Week Two

In Week Two, you want to cut back your dairy consumption (in addition to what you've already cut out in Week One). If you want dairy, try skim milk, nonfat yogurt or nonfat cheese. You will also totally wipe all fast-food out of your program. You also are going to add a fourth meal. Here's a schedule:

Meal One: Whole grain cereal (like Shredded Wheat or oatmeal) with skim milk, toast with jam, and four to five egg whites. (If you don't know how to do egg whites, I'll teach you how later.)

Meal Two (which will come three hours after first meal): Turkey sandwich with mustard, a baked potato with salsa sauce or yogurt or nonfat sour cream—but no butter or full-fat sour cream.

Meal Three: One portion of grilled chicken, a cup of rice, and a cup of a fibrous vegetable like broccoli.

Meal Four: A baked fish, salad, and pasta.

Remember that I'm only giving you examples of the food to eat. You can eat whatever proteins you want, for example, as long as you make sure that they are only the leanest of proteins. Also, in Week Two, you are allowed to eat two cheat meals.

Week Three

In addition to everything else we have reduced, in Week Three we are now going to reduce sugars and sweet fruits. Eliminate the alcohol and soft drinks totally. We're also adding a fifth meal.

> *Meal One*: Five egg whites, cereal with skim milk, two slices of dry toast (notice that we've cut out the jam).
>
> *Meal Two*: Grilled chicken with rice and a fibrous veggie.
>
> *Meal Three*: A meal similar to Meal Two.
>
> *Meal Four*: A white fish or chicken or very lean cut of red meat (remember, never let your meats be cooked with oil), a complex carb (potato or rice), and a salad with lemon or vinegar dressing.
>
> *Meal Five*: Same as Meal One.

This week, you get only one cheat meal. But try to make it a better cheat meal than usual. I want to introduce you to the concept of a "good cheat." If you want pizza as your cheat meal, then try it without cheese. If you want Mexican food, ask that the chips be removed from the table and replaced with corn tortillas.

Week Four

You are now going to reduce processed foods such as pastas, breads and cereal out of the program. You are going to try to eat out less (so you won't be subjected to the hidden fats and oils of restaurant food), and you're going to get into the habit of healthy cooking and bringing food with you to work so you can get your meals in every three hours.

In this week's meal plan, make sure to balance your proteins, carbs and fibrous vegetables at your meals (except the first one). It's now a sin to miss your fifth meal.

Meal One: Four to six egg whites and one bowl of oatmeal.

Meal Two: Chicken, rice and a fibrous vegetable.

Meal Three: Similar to Meal Two.

Meal Four: A meat, a complex carb, and a fibrous vegetable— similar to Meals Two and Three.

Meal Five: Same as Meal One.

You get one cheat meal this week.

Week Five

You're really at the advanced level of the North Program, because you're going to take those foods that you reduced in the previous weeks and now eliminate all of them. I also want you to try to reduce, if not eliminate, all red meat for the next two weeks. For your meal plan, eat exactly as Week Four.

Week Six

Congratulations. I know if you've been doing the program so far, you have seen tremendous change already. But believe it or not, you can still make more progress. Now, you must eliminate all cheating to the best of your ability. You must strip every ounce of excess fat from your diet. And in this streamlined, perfect week, your body's metabolism is going to be flying, burning up every-thing in sight. You're going to feel lean. You're also, quite frankly, going to feel hungry. You can't wait until that next meal. But, you cannot cheat this week. Instead, we're adding a sixth meal.

You might be asking, "Why eat six meals a day? Isn't five enough?" I'm not saying you have to eat the sixth meal. If it's late at night and you're tired or you're not hungry, skip it. You're not hurting the program. If you are in great need of losing weight, then you might also want to consider skipping it. But if you're on the program, and you want to gain muscle, then a small sixth meal is very important. Indeed, the sixth meal is a great boost in keeping the metabolism revved up. Here's a six-meal day for Week Six:

Meal One (around 7:00 a.m.): Oatmeal and four to six egg whites.

Meal Two: A small serving of a turkey breast, a cup of rice and a cup of broccoli.

Meal Three: A grilled chicken breast, a baked potato, a cup of corn and one fibrous vegetable.

Meal Four: Steamed fish, an order of beans, and a salad with lemon dressing.

Meal Five: Chicken, a serving of potato and a fibrous vegetable.

Meal Six (around 10:00 p.m.): The same as Meal One.

Do I Have to Stay At Week Six?

You should try to stay at this level as long as you can or until you get to your desired look where you are happy and comfortable.

But then, don't drop off for a week or two and go back to your old ways. Don't binge. Don't think you can give it all up for a month and come roaring right back. All I want you to do is just reintegrate certain foods that you cut out during those first six weeks. If you feel your body fat is coming back, then cut out those foods once again.

Once again, I'll tell you that it's okay to cheat. You are doomed to fail if you try to go through life depriving yourself of the foods you most enjoy and like to eat most frequently. But it's been my experience with clients that as they finally learn to eat correctly and as they develop a North Body, they don't want to return to their old greasy or fried foods. They lose the taste for them.

Also remember the extra benefit of higher metabolism. When you reach your desired goals with your body, you'll be able to cheat and still not store fat the way you did in the past. You'll be able to eat an extra cookie here and there because it will get burned up in your high-metabolism body. Just don't overdo it. Cheating is one thing. Bingeing is something else.

How Much To Eat in a Meal?

Quantities vary on the size of the person in the program. If you're a man over two hundred pounds, for example, you might want to go for six to eight egg whites in your first meal and a large chicken breast in your other meals. If you're a woman under one hundred and twenty pounds, you'll probably want to drop to three to five egg whites and eat a much smaller chicken breast.

You want your complex carb and fibrous vegetable to be about one cup per serving (a cup-and-a-half if you're a larger man). A cup of food, for all you men who do not have measuring cups in your house, is about the amount of food you can put in a regular-sized coffee cup.

You want your meat to be between three and six ounces. Again for all you previously mentioned brilliant men, an ounce is about two full bites of meat put into the average-sized mouth. A three-ounce portion of meat is about the size of a pack of playing cards.

Above all, you have to listen to your body. Eat moderately at all times, but enough to get satisfied. However, there is a great difference between "satisfied" and "full." If you're trying to gauge how much to eat, why don't you stop about halfway through a meal, put down your silverware, and ask, "How hungry am I right now? How much more do I need to eat?"

And just in case you're slipping back into that old destructive thought pattern, don't worry about calories. You've just done a 180-degree turnaround on your eating. Considering that you're now eating only good foods, it will undoubtedly be better for you to eat more than what you were eating in the past.

At the beginning of this program, you may not crave four to five meals a day, but after doing this program for a couple of weeks, you won't be able to go more than two or three hours without eating a meal. And when you have an appetite, that's a very good sign.

Your Body Type

All of you will move at a different pace in the North eating program, and you need to know the reason for your pace has a lot to do with your body type. Depending on your body type, some of you will have to be more careful about cheating; others will find you can cheat a little more; some of you might have to be cognizant of keeping your portions small; and some might be able to eat liberally. But don't get discouraged. The North Program works for all of you. There are three types of bodies:

The Mesomorph. These are naturally muscular humans who can do minimal exercise and still have great bodies. They respond easily to training—Bo Jackson, Arnold Schwarzenegger, Chris Evert, Martina Navratilova and Herschel Walker are all mesomorphs—and they don't have to be fanatical about my eating program.

But a word of warning to you mesomorphs out there: Even though it all comes easily to you now, you can still fall prey to the big gut or thunder thighs. You need to know that later in life, you are always the hardest person to get back in shape or to get back on a good eating program, because you've been so accustomed to everything coming so easily. The North Program is perfect for you because it gives you a healthy eating program, not a "diet," which you would ignore anyway.

The Ectomorph. Michael Jackson is an ectomorph. So is Don Knotts and Twiggy. Ectomorphs tend to be tall and skinny, with stringy, longer limbs. In sports, they tend to excel at endurance activities such as marathon running and cycling. If you're an ectomorph, you sometimes think you can eat whatever you want without putting on weight. Indeed, you can get away with taking in a little more fat and sugar. But that doesn't mean you should. To build a better body, you need to increase your amount of protein and carbohydrates. You don't want to gain fat; you want to gain quality muscle, which enhances body contours. You also need to make sure to eat more than you think you need. Why? Because right now, when you think you're eating a lot, you're probably not. You're still eating half of what a mesomorph eats. The North eating plan is perfect for you because it will make you get the right number of meals in, leading you to a more beautiful, shapelier body.

The Endomorph. The person who tends to be on the round side. Compared to an ectomorph, an endomorph puts on weight very easily. If you're an endomorph, you'll probably need to do longer aerobics to keep your fat down. But you'll also need to follow the North meal plan more carefully. With your bigger appetite, you have to be careful about eating too much food in one meal. You also have to be more concerned with missing meals—because when you miss meals, you'll have the tendency to want to binge.

Gaining More Weight, or Losing More Weight?

For both ectomorphs and endomorphs, there are going to be times, as you progress in the North Program, when you might have to tinker with your meal plans.

It you want to reduce weight on the North meal plan, then perhaps you should cut out egg whites on your first meal and carbohydrates on your last meal to reduce more weight. Gradually, you might want to shave your portion sizes. If you want to use the North Program for weight gain, then just add a couple of more carbohydrates like whole-grain breads and pastas to your meals to gain weight. If you're an ectomorph, you probably burn energy in overdrive already, so more carbohydrates will keep the body from eating into its muscle. Maybe add a protein drink.

What If I Still Want to Overeat?

In the unlikely case that you do keep eating too much and overloading your system, even in a six-meal-a-day plan, it's time for some old-fashioned willpower. I have four suggestions:

1. Simply slow your eating pace at mealtimes. I know this is hard—when I'm hungry, I'm a wolf. But as you eat, your blood sugar level rises, which causes insulin to be released. When insulin levels reach a certain point, a satiety or "full" signal is sent to the brain. For most of us, this takes about twenty minutes from the time we take our first bite of food. Therefore, fast eating encourages overeating.

2. To aid in controlling your portion sizes, if you're an overeater, then don't eat from your serving dishes or the containers you keep your food in. Put your portions on a plate and then put the rest of the food away before you eat. If you're at a restaurant, immediately have the waiter remove any crackers or bread he puts out before a meal. Don't give yourself the opportunity to nibble.

3. I hate lots of diet rules, because they can feel tyrannical; you're always being told to watch yourself. But here's one rule that does work: When you watch television, don't go into the kitchen during a commercial. Get up and walk anywhere except toward your refrigerator. Watching television makes a lot of people restless, and too many people interpret that restlessness as hunger.

4. As nutritionist Keith Klein says, make "good-bad" choices. Instead of a Dove Bar, have a nonfat yogurt. Eat fat-free chips instead of greasy potato chips. Try air-popped popcorn instead of buttered popcorn.

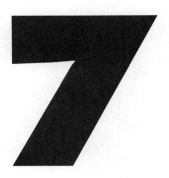

Fat Free for Life

The Foods You Must Have—and
the Foods to Throw Away

know all of you have made some attempts in the past to eat the right foods. It's okay, you can tell me—Uncle Larry. You're not doing too good a job at it, are you? I know that a Gallup poll says 76 percent of Americans say that they watch their diet to reduce fat. Americans consume 45 percent more lard and shortening than they did five years ago. The number of customers at fast-food restaurants has gone up. Americans overall eat nine pounds more sugar and other sweeteners a year and a pound more chocolate than they did in 1986. Americans, in fact, are eating two pounds more snack food each year.

This is, in all honesty, a disaster. Despite the loads of information that has been publicized about proper eating in the last decade, we're still succumbing to bad food.

We think we're getting around our bad food habits by listening to the teases of food manufacturers who promise us low-fat products that really add up to inconsequential caloric savings. We buy lots of what we think are nonfat desserts at the grocery store, neglecting to see on the label how much sugar those desserts have.

I know your entire North Program is going to fail if you don't clear the fattening foods out of your life. You too must realize—now that you've learned the principles of the eating program—that you can't be around such foods, especially as you get started. If you do, you'll obviously be tempted to eat them.

So I'm going to make this easy for you.

Get out a big garbage bag. Get a huge one.

Now take it into the kitchen and get ready to work.

I want you to throw out everything that's fattening, from potato chips in the pantry to ice cream in the freezer to mayonnaise in the refrigerator. If you can't bear to throw them away, give them away. But get them out of your house!

On the following pages is a list of things I never want in your kitchen again. Photocopy this list and tape it to your refrigerator next to the list on good foods to eat. Snack proof your shelves. You have to keep a kitchen that encourages only proper eating.

The Be-Careful List

There are enough bad foods out there that I could fill up this book naming them all, but this list should get you started:

Bacon

Nuts and seeds

Sausage

Dark meat chicken and turkey

Hot dogs and cold cuts

Tamales

Corny dogs

Fish sticks

Frozen waffles

Pancake mixes

Store-bought bread, white or wheat

Butter and margarine

Frozen juices

Candy

Chocolate syrup

Ice cream

Cool Whip

Pies

Pizzas

All chips and crackers

Coconut

Avocados

Pastries and cakes

All milk, except skim

Cream

Sour cream

Cottage cheese

Biscuits

Pudding

Peanut butter

Olives

Jellies and jams

Ketchup

Croutons

Salad dressings and mayonnaise

Cooking oils

Cooking sprays

Beef Jerky

Sardines

Canned fruit

Soft drinks and sodas

Boxed cereals

White flour

Sugar

Non dairy creamers

So, what does your empty kitchen look like? Pretty stark, right? Well, grab your car keys. Eating right begins at the supermarket— meaning that if you put the right foods in your shopping cart, you will almost certainly put the right nutrients in your body. Why, for example, do you eat those three doughnuts at the end of the night?

Because you bought them at the grocery store, you big dummy. What you need is a new shopping list. Let me give you a tour of your local supermarket, department by department, and show you exactly what you should buy.

The Shopping List
Meat Department

1. Deboned, skinless white meat chicken and turkey. Small chickens are leaner than large ones and turkey breast is leaner than chicken. Dark meat chicken is 40 percent fat, while white meat chicken is 6 percent fat. Always remove the skin from turkey and chicken. A full chicken, with flesh and skin, is 50 percent fat calories.
2. Sirloin, eye of round and round steak are the leanest cuts of beef.
3. Pork center tenderloin.
4. White fish like cod, flounder, haddock, scrod, halibut, shrimp, mussels, lobster and crab meat are the least fatty fish. (To give you an idea of what a nonwhite fish is like, salmon has six grams of fat for every three ounces.)
5. Just in case you're tempted, hot dogs, pork lunch meats, and ground beef are over 50 percent in fat. Even though turkey and chicken franks are proclaimed as lower fat than a beef frank, they still contain eight to eleven grams of fat each.
6. Venison
7. Turkey Tenderloin

Produce

1. Your best fruits (meaning less in sugar than the highly sweet fruits) are fresh strawberries, apples, pears and berries. Running in second place, but still okay, are grapefruit, cantaloupe, mangos, tangerines, oranges, honeydew, papayas, plums, and nectarines. Fruits like bananas, pine-

apples, peaches, grapes and watermelon are high in sugar, but eating a piece of this fruit for a snack or as part of a meal isn't going to hurt your program. (Just don't make the mistake of having a piece of fruit and calling it a meal, or a meal made up only of fruit. You'll overload your body with sugar that could easily turn into fat.) Definitely avoid avocados (one avocado is thirty-six grams fat) and all dried fruit like raisins (which has 210 calories per half cup).

2. Best fresh vegetables are carrots, spinach, peppers, cucumbers, onions, mushrooms, squash, lettuce, asparagus, celery, tomatoes, garlic, cabbage, broccoli, baking potatoes, sweet potatoes, corn, green beans, yams, zucchini, tomatoes, cauliflower, eggplant and Brussels sprouts.

3. Best beans and peas are red beans, kidney beans, black beans, pinto beans, black eyed peas, sweet peas and green peas.

4. Grains are brown rice, basmati rice, wild rice, oats, wheat berries, couscous, corn, barley, buckwheat grouts, brown rice, millet, bulgur, whole corn grits and triticale. (They can all be cooked like a rice pilaf, added to soups or eaten as is.)

Dairy

1. Skim milk
2. Nonfat sour cream and nonfat yogurt
3. Eggs
4. Nonfat cheese
5. Feta cheese, farmers' cheese and low-fat cottage cheese are your lowest fat cheeses. Not regular cottage cheese? Sorry, no. It is not a good "diet food" as your mother told you. It's got five grams of fat per half-cup.

Dressings and Sauces
1. Tabasco
2. Picante sauce
3. Yellow mustard and Dijon mustard
4. Seasoned vinegars, balsamic and wine vinegars (If you use them on your salads and vegetables, after a while you won't even miss the oil.)
5. Weight Watchers ketchup
6. KC Masterpiece Barbecue Sauce (very low in fat)

Canned Foods
1. Tuna packed in water
2. White meat chicken packed in water
3. Chicken broth
4. Canned beans (without fat or sugar)
5. Canned tomato paste
6. Canned fat-free sauces
7. Canned white meat turkey and chicken

Freezer Case
1. Frozen egg substitutes
2. Frozen vegetables
3. Frozen berries

Juices
1. Lemon juice
2. Lime juice
3. Gatorade Light

Chips/Snacks
1. Baked low-fat or nonfat corn tortilla chips
2. Nonfat potato chips
3. Pretzels have less fat than chips, but are still not recommended.

4. Popcorn, as long as it's air-popped and not prepared with cooking oil. "Natural flavored popcorn" usually has no less fat than butter-flavored.

Cereals/Breads

1. Oatmeal
2. Cream of wheat or shredded wheat
3. Grits
4. Unprocessed whole-grain bread

Seasonings

Chili powder, cilantro, cloves, dill weed, garlic, marjoram, parsley, tarragon, Italian herbs, mustard seed, onion powder, minced onion, lemon peel, orange peel, black pepper, cayenne pepper, red pepper, poultry seasoning, Molly McButter, Butter Buds, cinnamon, cumin, oregano, paprika, rosemary, thyme.

Other Low-fat and Nonfat Items

These days, you can get just about anything—nonfat mayo, nonfat dressings, nonfat sour cream, nonfat soups, nonfat crackers—and they all are fairly good. If you eat too many fat-free foods, which are often high in sugar, you won't lose weight because you're taking in so many empty calories. You're also robbing yourself with artificially flavored fat-free foods of vital nutrients that can be found in naturally fat-free foods. Remember, low-fat desserts are lower in fat, but they are still junk.

Watch out, as well, for frozen diet dinners that claim to be less than three hundred calories. Still, they are high in fat calories. One frozen diet dinner I saw had 280 calories, but 117 of them came from fat. That means almost half of the dish is fat calories.

What nonfat desserts do is keep you in the habit of looking for the taste of fatty-type foods. You have to hate fatty foods.

Special Reminders

1. *Read the labels.* You can't trust an item just because it says "low fat." That just means it's lower in fat than the original item, but by how much? Thankfully, the industry is finally changing its labeling: by mid-1994, according to new federal regulations, a food can't be labeled as "low fat" unless there are only three grams of fat in every fifty grams of that particular food. But you still need when reading labels to look for anything ending in "ose," like fructose. That means it's a sugar. You also must pay attention to the serving size. Don't make the mistake of thinking the whole package or can is one serving. This is one of the top mistakes people make. One package may actually contain ten or more servings.

2. *Vitamins.* Because you're cutting out such things as dairy and fruits that you might be accustomed to eating, you might, as an insurance policy—as a supplement to your new eating program—buy any generic brand of multivitamin tablet and a multimineral tablet. If you wish, add a vitamin C tablet. If you are really eating the perfect nonfat diet, then you might want to buy "essential fatty acid" tablets, taking four to six a day, just to make sure you are getting the essential fat your body needs. Do not be tempted by fat-burning pills: they burn fat off the liver but they don't rid your body of fat. There is no over-the-counter fat-burning supplement that can truly burn body weight off your body. Remember, the most powerful health supplement is your mind.

3. *Health Foods.* Foods that claim they are "All Natural Health Foods" can be the most fat-laden substances in the grocery store. Six ounces of tofu has a whopping sixteen grams of fat. Natural peanut butter has more fat than regular peanut butter. All-natural potato chips and granola are ridiculously full of fat.

A one-ounce serving of that health store favorite, sunflower seeds, contains fifteen grams of fat.

4. *Water.* Don't forget water, the cheapest thing you'll get on the North Program. A woman's body is 55-65 percent water. A man's is 65-75 percent water. And the water in your bodies has to be replenished constantly. The standard rule—drink eight glasses of water a day—is very important because water aids digestion, cleans out the body, helps metabolize fat, and gives you the psychological feeling that you're full. (If you're really hungry and it's not time for your meal yet, drink a glass of water and see what happens.)

5. *Sugar.* Many of you still have lots of questions about how much sugar you can take in, since sugar technically has no fat. But sugar, in excess, will put body fat on. Sugar gets a harmful cycle going in your body. If you take in a large amount of sugar, like a candy bar, your body has a sugar high that gives you a false sense of energy. When the sugar high subsides, you feel listless, and so psychologically you demand a bigger high—which means you consume even more sugar.

Here's the problem. When you take in sugar, it goes right into the bloodstream. Sugar in the bloodstream is carried to the fat stores. That, in turn, makes your pancreas release insulin to counteract the sugar. The insulin triggers those mechanisms in the body that collect fat. Boom! Greedily, the fat cells will take in that sugar and turn it to more fat. The sad truth is, people who eat too much sugar will store it as fat. Even if you eat something low in fat but high in sugar, you will still gain weight.

Also, don't be fooled by the words "natural sugar." All sugar is natural. And all sugar is refined. Brown sugar, which a lot of people think is better for them, is 99 percent refined, only 1 percent removed from white table sugar.

Eating Out

When I tell you to clean the bad food from your refrigerator and pantries, and then bring in the good food from your neighborhood grocery store, I know I am hitting only part of the equation. It would be easy to eat right if you locked yourself in your house with the proper foods. But most Americans eat away from home an average of four times a week (I often do that four times a day!), and Americans are spending 40 percent of their monthly food budgets at restaurants.

Obviously, if you can't stay on the North Program when you're at a restaurant, then you're in trouble once again.

Ten years ago, it would have been nearly impossible to stay on the North Program if you ate out. But now, even some fast-food restaurants are serving fresh salad and baked potatoes. You can get steamed vegetables at other restaurants. Yes, we are improving. There are several restaurants in Dallas serving my North Plate, the perfectly balanced meal which I'll tell you about later.

But beware. Most restaurants still serve you foods with hidden fats—and these are the ones advertising "healthy food." Other restaurants routinely drown their food in fat, butter and oils. They will marinate chicken breasts in oil or butter which soaks into the meat. Rice is cooked with butter and oil; most vegetables have added butter. So if you are going to survive out there in the cruel world, then you'd better know how to "special order" in restaurants.

This chapter is one of the most crucial in the whole book. Many of you eat very well at home, but when you go to a restaurant you don't try to cut out fat because you don't think you can control your meals. I'm going to teach you that you can.

Talking to Your Waiter

I am amazed to watch hard-driving businessmen—tough negotiators at the conference table—act completely passive at a dining table. They might work up the courage to ask what kind of oil is used to cook their entree, and if told that it's hydrogenated vegetable oil, they'll say, "Well, um, okay."

No, it's not okay. You've got to learn to look the waiter in the eye and say, "Please, this is very important. Make sure my chicken is cooked in no oil or butter. Period." Right now, in the privacy or your room, take a deep breath and say the following: "Sir (or Ma'am), I cannot have any sauces put on my food." There, that wasn't hard, was it?

I know one man who says to his wait person, "Listen, I have a heart condition, and if there's any oil in my food, I can guarantee you I'm going to have cardiac arrest right here on the floor." You don't have to go that far, of course. But what is wrong with being firm with your waiter, and letting him know that it's not okay to cook your food with even a small amount of fat, and that if your food is not prepared as you asked, you'll send it back?

One good way to beat the psychological barrier is to call the restaurant in advance and ask about low-fat, non-oil dishes you could order that evening. Or when you go into a restaurant, tell your waiter in advance that you are on a restrictive low-fat diet. Tell him politely that you're sorry to disappoint the chef (after all, if you're a chef trained to make veal parmesan, wouldn't you be a little hurt if an order came in for a straight piece of chicken?), but then ask the waiter if he or she can accommodate you. Of course, you'll be told yes. The fact is that restaurants are becoming more aware of the health-conscious customer. If you ask in a pleasant voice about special requests, and if you say you'll take good care of the waiter with a gratuity, then you'll get what you want.

Know What You're Doing

But if you go into a restaurant wanting low-fat food, you have to be a little educated. You can't go into an Italian restaurant and order a steaming plate of creamy topped pasta and say, "and make that low fat." No chef can take the cheese out of fettucine Alfredo.

But the waiter is going to respect you more if you say you want pasta dressed only in garlic with a splash of vinegar, or perhaps with a little wine and tomato. When you order fish or chicken, ask for it grilled without oil or butter (you can also ask for it to be cooked with lemon or lime juice). That way, if your meat shows up with a slick of butter covering it, you can boldly demand that it be taken back.

Or here's another common mistake. Instead of ordering an omelet for breakfast, you proudly, as a fledgling North Program follower, ask for an egg white omelet. You didn't go far enough. You'll get the egg whites, but the omelet has been cooked in butter and covered with cheese. You're still looking at a thirty-fat-gram omelet—a massive piece of fat. Be more specific. Say: "I would like an egg white omelet without cheese and prepared with no butter or oil." That brings your omelet down to zero fat grams. Here's some other things to try and watch for in restaurants:

1. Ask for vegetables that are steamed, boiled or sautéed in water only.

2. Don't order any soups that are cream or meat based. That's a usual indication of high fat.

3. Ask the waiter if the chef blanches food in oil. This is the process where the cooks (especially at Chinese restaurants) put vegetables into scalding high-fat oil to cleanse or loosen the peel. Tell the waiter you don't want your food all blanched.

4. Ask for all dressings and sauces on the side or request that they be omitted from your order altogether. If you do use them for flavoring, dip your fork in the dressing and then spear your food. That gives you enough of a taste. Don't do it the other way around, which is to spear your food first then dip it in the dressing. In that case, your food will be slathered with dressing. Lemon and vinegar are great substitutes for salad dressing.

5. Ask that any nuts and seeds be removed from your dishes.

6. Ask the waiter to remove any temptations from your table, such as butter, bread, crackers and chips. A roll with butter while you are waiting for your meal is an estimated 150 calories.

7. Be careful at the salad bars. Many offer high-fat choices such as bacon bits, cheese and croutons. Avoid all premade salads such as pasta and potato salads. They are loaded with mayonnaise and other fat.

8. Avoid, if possible, alcohol with your meal. That will make you overeat. If you do want a drink, try a wine spritzer (wine with soda), which has fewer calories than a glass of wine. Even if you drink a beer with no fat, the beer, loaded with sugar and calories, cuts down on your body's ability to burn fat.

9. Ask about side dishes that come with your meal. For example, if you order a turkey sandwich with mustard—a good selection—it might come on a plate heaped with potato chips and coleslaw. You will be tempted to dig into those foods too. Tell your waiter to keep them from your table.

10. Avoid the classic "Dieter's Plate" at restaurants. A typical sirloin patty, cottage cheese and tomato slices can be 70 percent fat.

11. Do not feel you must eat everything just because you paid for it. Remember that you usually will get larger portions at a restaurant than what you give yourself at home. Don't hesitate to share your food. But on the other hand, don't let your fellow diners talk you into sharing a dessert. Don't be intimidated. Ask for encouragement from them, bring up how great you feel since you have been on the program, and they won't pressure you.

The North Plate

The North Plate has become a popular meal at many Dallas restaurants—it usually consists of a grilled chicken breast, brown rice and broccoli—but you can put together a North Plate at any restaurant, even the greasiest hamburger joint.

Never forget that at each meal you're wanting a protein, a complex carb and a fibrous vegetable. Look the menu over very carefully to see what foods the restaurant has in its kitchen. Let's take the hamburger restaurant. They usually have lots of lettuce and tomatoes to dress out a hamburger. All right, there's your fibrous vegetable. They make French fries from a baked potato, so ask politely if they might have an extra baked potato lying around that you can have served plain. There's your complex carb. Usually, these restaurants also serve chicken sandwiches. If the chicken can be grilled without oil, get it plain (no bread or mayonnaise), then pull off any skin or fat when it arrives. There's your protein.

Other Restaurants

I know some people who don't look at a menu when they walk into a restaurant because they don't want to be tempted. They ask for a grilled meat, a potato dish and a steamed vegetable. In fact, regardless of what style of restaurant you visit, there are some specific dishes you can look for.

French: You can ask for an egg-white omelet, filet of sole, poached sea bass, trout or bay scallops, or grilled meat in wine sauce. There will usually be a standard salad you can get without dressing. If it's a spinach salad, ask that no bacon or egg be added. Avoid Hollandaise or any sauce based in cream. Avoid sautéed dishes at French restaurants unless the food is sautéed in water. Avoid duck and paté.

Italian: Look for a vegetable plate with no sauce, meatless pasta with oil-free marinara sauce or wine sauce, or a vegetarian pizza with no cheese and no added oil on the crust. Avoid any cream sauces and fatty meats like prosciutto. Avoid Parmesan cheese. Avoid breaded veal, or breaded vegetables and white breads. Watch out for olive oil, which many restaurants tend to overuse.

Plain pasta might seem like a good choice, but it often has oil in the boiling pot and when rinsed, the oil stays on the pasta.

Mexican: Look for fresh fish marinated in lime sauce with beans and rice. You can order unfried corn tortillas, chicken enchiladas without the creamy sauce, or chicken fajitas grilled in lemon or lime juice instead of oil. Avoid cheese, chips, sour cream, guacamole and refried beans (ask for whole beans instead). It's very easy to do a North Plate at a Mexican restaurant: Order grilled chicken with no oil, corn tortillas (instead of higher fat flour tortillas), rice instead of refried beans, pico de gallo instead of guacamole, and no cheese. Have the lettuce, tomato and onion on the side.

Chinese: Go for Moo Goo Gai Pan without sauce. Ask for any fresh or steamed vegetables. Make sure only white meat chicken is used in dishes. Ask that the dishes be stir fried without oil or salt and that they be cooked in broth or water. Choose the dishes that come with sliced meat rather than diced meat (diced often has fatter cuts). Order steamed rice, not fried. And avoid the egg rolls, any batter-fried item, any egg dishes and dishes loaded with nuts. Don't order beef or pork, and never order the duck (a three-and-a-half ounce serving of Peking duck has thirty grams of fat).

Indian: You can find low-fat legumes, steamed vegetables, chicken or fish that has been marinated and roasted without oil, and chutney adds a lot of flavor without adding fat.

Steak: At a steak restaurant, ask for a large dinner salad without cheese or croutons. Ask for a baked potato with yogurt or Dijon mustard. And most of these restaurants offer a grilled chicken on the menu; ask that all the fat be trimmed and no oil be used in preparation. You usually can also find shrimp.

Fast Food: There is very little nutritional value in fast food. The whole concept goes against every nutritional principle. All fast foods supply you with very high-calorie foods that are basically sugar and fat, and lack any fiber or vitamins. Don't think chicken is better than hamburgers. A single fried chicken nugget is going to have an entire tablespoon of mostly saturated fat. Fast-food chicken sandwiches have as much fat as hamburgers. Don't think you can buy fried chicken, and peel off the skin and get good chicken. That piece of chicken has been so soaked in oil that the fat has seeped down into the bone. If you must, try to go vegetarian in a fast food restaurant. Get the lettuce and tomato and look for a baked potato.

Eating on the Road

There will be times when you are out of town and you can't find a restaurant that looks like it could serve your needs. My suggestion is that it's just as convenient to stop at a local grocery store, get four to five ounces of sliced, salt-free turkey, order a baked potato from the deli, get some carrots and a green apple from the produce department—and you've got a meal.

If you are traveling by car, you can prepare a basket or cooler of food, including bagels, fresh sliced turkey, raw vegetables, apples and water. You can bring along such food as spices, Butter Buds, oatmeal, instant rice, tuna, water, canned veggies, and a can opener. Presto. You've got meals. If you are traveling by plane, request low-fat meals when you book your reservations. At your hotel, you can ask for a portable microwave or small refrigerator, then make a quick trip to the grocery store—and you can get in a meal or two at your hotel room without going through the hassle of looking for an adequate restaurant. There are plenty of ways to be creative. All you need is commitment.

Cooking 101, the North Method

I know you're laughing. Larry North, the muscle head, teaches *you* how to cook. Give me a break. Isn't that about the same as Julia Child teaching you to lift weights?

Yes, I really have the guts to write a chapter about the joy of cooking, Larry North style. I've learned there are still a lot of people out there in this culinary age who don't have a clue how to do some basic meals—how to crack open an egg, or how to make healthy grilled chicken, or how to make brown rice. I definitely know my words are hitting home with the bachelors who are so intimidated by cookbooks that they've never gotten around to turning on the stove. I also know there are many women who have been so busy conducting their lives that they never learned to cook. And now they are too embarrassed to ask someone what to do.

Welcome, all of you, to my kitchen. The truth is that healthy low-fat cooking has never been easier. It is not time consuming, and it doesn't take extra effort. In the back of this book you'll get a variety of truly delicious recipes for low-fat or nonfat dishes.

But there's no question that all of you need to be reminded of some of the basic, simple things to do to prepare the right foods. I'm not going to be fancy (oh, wow, that's a surprise—no Larry Soufflé!). But who really has the time for spending two or three hours to cook one meal? You need to know how to get the right food—and lots of it—on the table.

The Need to "Pre-Prepare"

The key to the North eating program—and I'm not exaggerating for a second—is that you must prepare large quantities of food. If you don't have plenty of foods ready to eat—fibrous vegetables, complex carbs and proteins—you'll start missing meals. You'll also start driving yourself crazy, considering how you're going to be eating so frequently from now on, if you don't have preprepared food. I guarantee you won't be able to cook for each meal. You'll be so behind you'll find yourself snacking on everything that's going to sabotage your program.

In a couple of hours, you can cook almost everything you'll need for a whole week. You need the regular array of pots and pans, some Tupperware containers and food storage bags, and you're ready.

I can pop a dozen chicken breasts on the grill, put ten baked potatoes in the oven, boil beans and steam vegetables on the stove—and I'm done in two hours. Corn, fish fillets, vegetables, salads, beans, peas, potatoes, rice, and chicken are just some of the foods I pre-prepare.

The food I will eat the first three days, I store in the refrigerator. The rest, I put in the freezer. I take that out to thaw the night before I'm going to need to eat it. I reheat a chicken breast, some brown rice and black-eyed peas, and I'm ready for a meal.

"Larry," you say with a disgusted look, "this is not what someone would call gourmet eating."

So what? Do *you* eat a magnificent meal every time you sit down at a table? I need small, frequent meals, and this is the best way I know to do it. Besides, I know I'm eating as nutritiously as possible. And in my world, that stands for a lot.

Your First Cooking Lesson

Okay, my students, get all your utensils out. Your wooden spoons, your pots, your skillets.

Uh-oh, you made your first mistake. Go out and purchase all nonstick cookware. That's Chef Larry's first big rule. Why is that, my earnest students? Because you don't want to use oil or butter when you cook. That's a huge no-no.

What about nonstick spray? Nonstick spray is nothing but oil in a can. If you look at the ingredients, you're basically getting vegetable oil. That means with one spray of your skillet you have just added six to seven extra grams of fat to your food.

Naughty, naughty.

All right. Let's move on. Make sure you have a stove, a refrigerator, a microwave. Remind yourself that if you catch the kitchen on fire, you should run for your life.

Just kidding. If your kitchen catches on fire, call the fire department first, then run for your life.

Cooking, A to Z

What I'm going to do is take you through a day of meals, showing you what you'll need to do to cook the basic foods you'll eat on the North Program.

A quick tip: If you're hungry while you're cooking, keep a glass of water close by. Reach for it instead of nibbling what you are preparing. Or, if desperate, chew sugarless gum. The act of chewing keeps your mouth busy.

Morning Foods

1. *Oatmeal.* I suggest using three-minute oatmeal because it tastes better. You can simply eat it dry or with skim milk. Or you can pour boiling water over your oatmeal in a bowl and eat. Or you can mix the oatmeal with tap water in a bowl and microwave it for a minute-and-a-half. Eat with such things as cinnamon, Butter Buds, nutmeg and berries.

2. *Hard-Boiled Eggs.* Bring water in a pot to a boil, gently drop in the eggs, and boil for ten to fifteen minutes. Here's a secret to peeling eggs, which no one does well. As soon as you pull a hot egg from the pot, hold it under cold running water while you peel. Of course, eat only the egg whites.

3. *Scrambled Egg Whites.* Crack the egg gently in half, but let nothing run out. And now you face the task of getting the egg white out while keeping the yellowed yolk in the egg. Holding the two halves of the cracked egg, pour the egg yolk from shell to shell and let all the egg white drip into a bowl. Then pour the egg white into a preheated nonstick skillet. Scramble the egg with a wooden, plastic or rubber utensil. Using a metal utensil with nonstick cookware will ruin the cookware.

4. *Egg-White Omelet.* Prechop your desired ingredients (onions, green peppers, tomatoes, precooked chicken breast, broccoli, etc.) and either precook them by microwaving or heating them on the stove (cooking the ingredients only in water, no

oils or butter). Then, pour your egg whites into a warm skillet, but do not scramble. Take a wooden spoon and gently make small incisions about an inch long in your omelet so the uncooked parts of the egg white can flow into the bottom of the skillet. When most of the eggs are cooked, cover your skillet. The steam will cook the remainder of the egg white. Don't leave the omelet unattended as it will take too long to cook. Uncover and gently loosen the entire perimeter of the omelet from the pan with a plastic spatula. Turn the heat off. Pour on your vegetable and chicken ingredients. Then gently fold the omelet in half, still keeping it in the skillet. Now, you must act like a real chef. Slide the omelet out of the skillet onto the plate—shout "voila!" in a French accent—and there you have it. If you mess up and break the omelet, then just mix it around in the skillet and you have—Voila!—scrambled eggs.

5. *Bagel.* Don't laugh. A lot of people don't know what to do. Slice it in half and stick the halves in the oven. Turn the knobs to "Broil." Broil until the halves are brown. You'll be surprised how good a plain-toasted bagel tastes.

Meats

Make sure, whatever meat you get, to trim off the skin and all visible fats before cooking.

1. *Baked Chicken or Fish.* Cover a baking sheet with foil, pre-heat the oven to 450 degrees. Place skinless chicken breast or fish on the sheet, spice it, then bake for as long as it takes. Advice to beginners: After fifteen minutes, cut a piece of the meat in the middle and check to see if it's cooked.

2. *Sautéed Chicken or Fish.* Put herbs and one cup of wine (you can add Dijon mustard or lemon juice to the wine) into a skillet. Place chicken or fish in skillet, cover, and simmer on low heat for fifteen minutes on each side.

3. *Grilled Chicken, Fish, or Lean Cuts of Beef.* Marinate your meat in any variety of nonfat liquids—nonfat chicken broth with spices, any sort of citrus juices, fat-free barbecue sauce, or low-sodium soy sauce with ginger and garlic—slap the meat on the grill for seven to ten minutes each side. Don't try to poke with a knife because it will release all the meat's juices. Now you're done.

4. *Broiled Chicken or Fish.* Preheat the broiler, cover a baking sheet with foil, spice your chicken or fish, and broil. This type of cooking is very fast, about five minutes a side, so after a few minutes, check to see if the meat is done, then flip it over when cooked.

5. *Turkey Breast.* Put a turkey breast in a Reynolds cooking bag and bake in the oven at 325 degrees. Cook for twenty minutes a pound. Add seasonings if you wish.

6. *Microwaved Fish.* This is surprisingly good. Buy a white filleted fish, rinse it, sprinkle lemon pepper over it, squeeze half a lemon on top. Place the fish on a plate, cover in plastic wrap, pop in the microwave for a couple of minutes—and serve.

Vegetables

1. *Beans.* Buy a bag of beans, rinse them in a strainer (a bowl with holes in it). Pour the beans into a bowl that is four times bigger than the amount of the beans (the beans will later expand). Cover in water and leave overnight. The next day, dump the water, rinse the beans again, put them in the pot, fill with water—and let them boil for ten minutes. Then let that cool completely. Dump the water again (this is the best technique to use to avoid digestive gas), rinse, fill the pot for the last time with water, bring the water to boil, then turn the heat down just to a tiny boil. Boil for one to two hours until the beans are soft. You can add seasonings such as liquid smoke,

garlic and onion. If you want to gamble, experiment with herbs like basil, oregano, chili powder and red pepper.

2. *Broccoli.* Hack off the bottom stalk part of the broccoli. Skinned broccoli stems are good and nutritious. Now, you can put the broccoli on a plate, wrap it in plastic, and microwave for two minutes or until the broccoli turns bright green (for best results, make sure the broccoli stem is facing the door). Or you can put the broccoli in a skillet with water, covered with a collapsible steamer. Cook on high for ten to twenty minutes. Don't put in too much water or the vitamins will leak away. Or you can stir fry broccoli by breaking the broccoli into mouth-sized pieces. Then chop up a couple of cloves of garlic. Heat up the skillet and put in two teaspoons of de-fatted chicken broth along with the garlic. Add the broccoli. Stir until it turns bright green.

3. *Corn.* Cook the same as broccoli, unless you want to boil it in a big pot of water for five minutes. Use Molly McButter or Butter Buds. But put on the butter substitutes while the corn is still steaming hot. It will end up tasting better.

4. *Carrots.* Slice carrots into coin-sized pieces, drop in a pot of water and cook for ten to fifteen minutes. To add flavor, add a tablespoon of maple syrup for each carrot.

5. *Brown Rice.* Bring a pot of water to a boil and drop in your brown rice (for every cup of rice you put in, you need two cups of water). Cover the pot, and leave it for fifty-five minutes. You can cook in chicken broth instead of water. Or you can add a package of chicken noodle soup and give more taste to your rice. To a regular pot of rice, you can also add diced onions, bell peppers, cilantro, mushrooms, onions and white wine.

6. *Baking Potatoes.* Buy russet potatoes for baking. To bake, turn oven to 450 degrees, pierce the potatoes a couple of times, bake for forty-five minutes. If you bake your potatoes without foil, they'll come out a little more fluffy. Microwaving your

potatoes takes eight to ten minutes. Instead of butter, margarine or sour cream for toppings, try salsa, nonfat yogurt, nonfat butter substitutes and chives. Want to try Larry's Loaded Baked Potato? After you've baked your potato, take deli-sliced turkey, wrap it in a paper towel, pop it into the microwave on high for a few minutes. Then crumble the turkey, which now tastes like bacon bits, over the potato, add a butter substitute, nonfat cheese, nonfat sour cream, green onions or chives. Voila! C'est magnifique.

7. *New Potatoes.* Cut your new potatoes into chunks, put them in a pot of water, boil at high or medium for twenty minutes or until soft. Ready to serve, or you can create a potato salad using nonfat mayonnaise, green onion, pepper, and dill.

8. *Larry Fries.* After microwaving, boiling or baking a potato (the potato does not have to be fully cooked), shave the potato into thin pieces. Cover a cookie sheet with foil and lay out the pieces. After putting the potato slices on the foil, sprinkle with spices like garlic powder, paprika, salt and pepper. Put the potato slices in oven and broil until brown and puffy. Flip them over with spatula. Broil some more. Pull out and you have perfect, nonfat fries.

9. *Tossed Salad.* Use a combination of lettuces, shred carrots in a grater, slice a bell pepper, put in any fresh raw vegetables you want (you want raw vegetables every day for good nutrients). For a new kind of low-fat dressing, buy a vinaigrette dressing, pour out all the oil on top and use what's on the bottom. Or try vinegar Dijon mustard mixed with honey.

10. *Tuna Salad.* To make a delicious tuna salad, get water-packed tuna and fat-free mayonnaise. Put in onion, celery and egg whites. If you're a gambler, add Dijon mustard, vinegar, cilantro, tomatoes and onion.

And so, my eager cooking students, now that you have your certificate from the famous Larry North Cooking School (and really, that was pretty simple, wasn't it?), I'm sure you're ready to go out and throw a huge dinner party for all your friends. In fact, *in the appendix*, I've provided a variety of other recipes for you to try that are perfect for the North Program.

At this point in the book, you should be very proud of yourself. You have learned how to eat, how to spread out your meals, how to order your meals, and how to cook them.

Commit yourself now to this meal program for the next six weeks. Watch what happens to your body. I promise you: You will never want to go back to your old foods again.

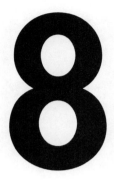

True Aerobics

The Foundation
for Your Better Body

ver the years, I've heard great excuses from you about why you can't work out. I don't make fun of you. I don't need to. I know when you say such things to me that you already know you are making excuses. You already know there is only one reason why you are not getting in shape. It's because you have chosen not to do so. I know you all are busy in your lives and careers, but I also know you have forty-five minutes a day each week where you are going to sit at home and watch television or leaf through a magazine. Hey, why don't you watch television or leaf through that magazine while riding a stationary bike? Why can't you take time out for a brisk walk?

When it comes to an aerobics program in your life, that's all I'm going to ask for—ever! And that's all you ever need. You never again have to believe that you must exercise as quickly as possible and as hard as possible until you drop. The glory of true aerobic activity is that you're better off precisely if you don't do that. If you work out longer with less intensity, then you will burn proportionately more calories that come from your body fat. And you also keep your body burning calories at a higher level after your body is at rest.

After reading this book, set up time to do a very basic aerobics program. Here, perhaps for the first time in your life, you're being told that it's better for you to work out with less intensity. You're being told that you're going to get a better fat burn if you do not go

full speed. There might be times when you'll want to do high intensity work to improve your cardiovascular fitness. But remember
what true fat-burning aerobics is all about. The number of calories
your body burns is related to the total amount of distance covered.
Thus, walking for an hour is better for you than running for twenty
minutes, assuming you cover a greater distance in that hour of
walking.

The Aerobics Secret

Still confused? It's time for another quickie science lesson.

If you do an aerobic exercise for a certain amount of time, your
body will start to run out of its available supply of glucose. It needs
other fuel to turn into glucose. It begins looking around for an
alternative fuel supply.

So far, so good. All you need to do is get your body to use its own
fat cells for fuel. If you can do that, then you lose body fat.

But here's the catch. If you train in such a way where you send
your body into "oxygen debt"—where you are panting for breath—
you stop burning fat. The oxygen debt builds up something called
lactic acid—and that acid inhibits the release of fatty acids to be
burned as fuel. You probably—and mistakenly—believe that when
you do very intense exercise at a very peak level, you are burning
pure fat. The scientific fact is, however, that you can only burn fat
one way—doing moderate exercise of long, steady duration. In
other words, to get the fat burned, you must slow down!

When you do the kind of exercise that puts you in oxygen debt,
you are no longer doing aerobics. You're doing something called
anaerobic exercise—exercise so demanding that your heart and
lungs are unable to supply enough oxygen. Most aerobics classes
you have taken in your life should be called "anaerobic classes."

"Wait, Larry," you say, "this can't be true. If I work out at a
strenuous level, surely I'm burning calories faster than if I take a
walk around the park."

Yes, you are. But don't forget that burning a lot of calories does not mean you're burning a lot of fat calories. You lose fat in ounces, not in pounds. When you are burning calories so quickly, you are losing something other than fat—your body is getting its energy and burning calories from your precious muscle. You want to learn to burn fat as efficiently as possible.

So, we're back to my basic exercise theory. Less is best. It's not who trains the hardest, but who trains the smartest.

How To Do It

I gauge a good aerobics programs on the following three factors: (1) frequency—how many times you do your aerobics, (2) duration—how long each session lasts, and (3) intensity—the least important of the three.

So what is intensity if it's not an all-out, sweat-and-grunt workout? Here's the North definition: during the entire time you do an aerobic exercise, you should be able to carry on a conversation. To see if you're doing the right level of exercise, just see if you can talk to someone at any point during your aerobics. If you can't, if you are breathing too heavily, then you're too intense.

That means to walk. Or get on the stationary cycle and enjoy yourself. Or do a light jog without feeling guilty that you should really be doing big-time long distance running. As your body gets more and more in shape through these exercises, then you will gradually increase your intensity level by going a little bit faster. But you will never, ever want to go fast enough to lose your breath. The goal of aerobics is not to exhaust you, but to invigorate you.

Frequency and Duration

There is only one price to pay for the perfect aerobics program—time. The longer you train, the more fat you burn. Basically, you want to spend between thirty to sixty minutes, three to five times a week, doing aerobics. You can do a lot more than that, of course.

If you went sixty minutes a day five times a week, you would be at your fat-burning best. Perhaps, as you get into the program and decide you need to reduce more weight, that's exactly what you're going to have to do.

But first, do the best you can. If you are out of shape and can't go thirty minutes straight, then break it up. Go fifteen minutes at a time; go ten minutes at a time if you have to. Do some of it in the morning and some in the evening. But get your aerobics in. As I said, frequency and duration are of top priority. When you go a steady, long pace, your body will continue to release energy by burning calories long after all of your physical activity has ceased.

A word of caution. Please, don't ever work at aerobics so hard that you feel your muscles ache. This is another myth about what aerobics is supposed to do. You don't want to wear down your muscles in aerobics. That's what the weight training is going to be for. You are in a multifaceted fitness program—eating, aerobics and weight training. Don't try to make one part of your program do everything for you.

What To Do

A lot of you just getting started rush up to me and ask, "Larry, what should I buy? A rowing machine? A stair climber? A cross country ski machine?" And I think, while your motives are good, you're missing the point.

First, all you have to do is walk. If you haven't been active for a long time, you need to start a consistent walking program. It will give you all the benefits, for now, of any machine. Take long walks, aiming to stride at a steady rate—nothing rigorous, but not a casual strolling pace.

According to the latest exercise studies, walking has more exercise potential than we have ever believed. Dr. Kenneth Cooper, the man who used to say that the more you ran the better off you'd be, now says that people should walk more and run less.

When you walk, you are not—as you do in running—bringing your entire body weight crashing down on each foot as it hits the pavement. You're not shocking your body with each step. Walking can produce an injury-free, stress-free activity.

There is one other aerobic exercise you might want to do right off as well—the stationary cycle. I say this because you can get a decent one starting at $300, and because a good piece of indoor aerobics equipment is great to have on rainy or cold days—or at night if you get home too late to do a walk. If you've got a bike in your house, you'll be amazed at the number of opportunities you have to ride it.

The Activities

When you pick an aerobics activity, make sure it fits your skill level. Just because something is difficult to do doesn't mean it gives you a better fat-burning workout. Once again, remember to do your aerobics three to five times a week, thirty to sixty minutes each session. While you can do everything from cross country skiing to walking up and down the stairs of your office building, the key is to make sure you are pushing yourself enough to raise your heart rate, but not enough to exhaust you.

Here's a sampling of activities:

Walking/Running:
    Level: Beginner to advanced
    Potential Injury: The risk of injury is high only for heavy runners who overtrain.
    Tip: Whenever possible, run on softer surfaces, and wear top running shoes. It's not worth it to harm your ankles and knees for a cheap shoe.
    Cost: $50-$100 for a good pair of running or walking shoes.

Treadmill:

Level: Beginner to advanced

Potential injury: Almost none, as long as the treadmill is well built. It's a perfectly controlled environment.

Tip: Make sure to straddle the machine before you go on and then slow the treadmill down to a stop before hopping off.

Cost: The good ones start at $1,500.

Stair Climbers:

Level: Beginner to advanced

Potential Injury: Very low, because stair climbers require less knee bending than going up real stairs. Could be troublesome if you have bad knees.

Tip: Always lean slightly forward when walking on stairs. But keep back straight. Don't lean so much that you are putting most of your body weight on the hand rails. Only use the handrails for balance.

Cost: The cheapest start at $150, but expect to pay much more for a good one. Be wary of stair-stepper machines; they are usually not cost-effective.

Outdoor Cycling:

Level: Moderate to advanced

Potential Injury: Some strain on lower back if you ride very long periods of time. And there's always a chance for injury if you take a spill.

Tip: For best results, set your seat size so there's just a slight bend in the knee at the bottom of your pedaling. Always wear a helmet.

Cost: $100 for the cheapest brand of bike to beyond $2,000 for the most expensive.

Stationary Bike:

Level: Beginner to advanced

Potential injury: Almost nonexistent unless you have bad knees.

Tip: Make sure the bike is sturdy and does not shift. A bike with a recumbent seat (reclining seat) burns more calories because it requires more muscle mass and is great for people with special needs such as pregnant women or people with bad backs.

Cost: $300 and up.

Cross Country Ski Simulator:

Level: Moderate to advanced

Potential injury: Slight strain on your back, but otherwise none.

Tip: It takes a lot of practice to get the movement down, so be patient. Once you do, you'll experience an effective, perfectly non-impact aerobic workout.

Cost: Good ones start at $400.

Swimming:

Level: Moderate to advanced

Potential injury: None. It's especially great for the disabled and the elderly, and people rehabilitating from injuries.

Tip: Even good swimmers can be helped by an instructor who will make their stroke smoother.

Cost: Minimal. Just find a pool at a facility such as a YMCA or YWCA, where fees are reasonable.

Warming Up

Many of you feel the need to do a lot of toe touching, leg stretching and trunk twisting before you exercise. You are making a mistake. You want to stretch at the end of a workout, when your muscles are warm. (And I will give you a series of stretching routines to do at the end of chapter 10.)

If you stretch your muscles when they are cold, you could tear muscle fibers, thus causing injury. I recommend that you literally shake yourself before you begin an aerobics workout. You want to loosely shake your hands, arms and legs to get the blood flowing. You want to lift your hands up and bring them down as if you're yawning. You are literally trying to wake up the body. Take some deep breaths to punch up your cardiovascular system. And then, when you start your aerobics activity, start slowly. Ease your body into the exercise. Don't ever try to shock your body into getting fit. You'll only be setting yourself up for the pain.

The Little Things

Have you heard the old saying—"Sitting is better than lying, standing is better than sitting?" Well, it's true. According to one study, there's a difference of about nine calories burned an hour between sitting quietly and standing quietly.

You can keep your metabolism higher by simply moving around more—walking, shopping, house cleaning, gardening and so on. In other words, mini-aerobics. There is evidence from the National Institutes of Health that in addition to regular aerobic exercise, body-fat loss can be enhanced by boosting all other activities throughout the day.

So I want you to take the extra step—literally. At the moment, it won't seem like much. But over a year's time, you will have burned off an amazing amount of extra calories. Plus, these mini-aerobics keep you in the right mind-set about staying fit. Here are some tips:

1. Consciously lengthen your stride every time you walk someplace. The effect will be to increase your pace as well as to naturally increase your energy output.
2. Where there are elevators, there have to be stairs. Climbing burns twice as many calories as walking on a level floor. So why ride one or two floors on an elevator when you can walk them?

3. Look for the nondriving opportunity. Walk or ride a bicycle instead of driving to a nearby location. Park your car in the most distant space in a parking lot instead of looking for a spot by the door.

4. Find ways to move around in your office. Walk to the more distant water cooler rather than the one by your desk. Walk to the corner mailbox. Start pacing around your office when you're thinking. At the least, don't sit for more than an hour without getting up and stretching for a few minutes.

5. Don't hesitate to participate in light recreational sports— shooting baskets, playing kickball or Ping-Pong with the kids, joining in a volleyball game. Somewhere inside you, fat is getting burned.

6. Always take a walk when you feel like napping. You'll discover you are more refreshed. Exercise has a better psychological effect than napping. It causes the release of endorphins that give you a kind of light euphoria (remember the famous "runner's high" we used to hear about?). Endorphins have been described as emotional tranquilizers that reduce anxiety. It is the best natural answer to stress that we possess.

Final Suggestions

1. It is a good idea eventually to "cross train"—varying your aerobics choices. One day walk, the next day cycle, and the next day you might want to take a swim. Cross training develops a more balanced state of fitness. It also helps reduce the risk of injury.

2. If you're going to do your aerobics training and weight training in the same day, it is better to do aerobics first before going to weights. Aerobics can be a wonderful way to warm up for the weight room. But if you are at a level where you do want to do a higher intensity aerobics workout, then do your weights first, so you can concentrate more on the weights and

not feel so tired.

3. Drink plenty of pure water before and after exercise. You're not going to get stomach cramps. Always keep replacing fluids while you're working out. Only out-of-date football coaches think you get in better shape by dehydrating yourself while exercising.

4. When should you exercise? I'm not one who says you have to work out exactly at the same time every day, but here's a suggestion. If you work out early in the morning, several things will happen. First, you will find you will want to eat right throughout the day because you got in a workout; you'll feel so good about yourself you won't want to blow it on a bad meal. Secondly, a morning workout means you don't have to worry about what might happen at the end of the day, when you might have to pick up a kid who's sick, or get somewhere for a dinner engagement. If you simply can't get in a morning workout, what about lunch? You don't need an hour to eat. You can eat one of the meals I've described in ten minutes. Then for the other forty minutes, why don't you put on a pair of tennis shoes and walk? Finally, the body thrives on consistency and regularity. If it's conditioned to work out at the same time each day, it will improve that much faster.

All right, we've made some big steps so far in the North Program. Now, go look at yourself. Take a long look. The change is beginning, your body is starting to take form. But I promise you, this is only the beginning. You're about to enter the weight room. Prepare yourself for the great transformation.

Weights for Life

Creating the Strong and Sexy Body

nce again, let me repeat—and repeat and repeat—myself. Muscle is the most valuable commodity to the body. Muscle is to your body what gold is to the economy. Think of your body. There are more than four hundred muscles there to keep your body firm—or to let it sag. Each muscle is composed of millions of tiny cells. There's no other way around it: to make those cells work, you've got to work them out. If you push those cells, you get more strength and more energy. If you put just a little resistance on your muscles, your body's contours, last seen in youth, start to return. You improve your posture and carriage. Your saggy skin tightens, your lungs provide more oxygen. Your bones, which have grown more brittle with age, actually gain more calcium and get stronger.

Weight training is the way a man can get the firm biceps and an upper back as wide as an eagle's wing span. Weight training is the way women get nice shapely legs and a small waist and tight hips. You can lose your thunder thighs, your saddlebag hips. Your love handles will remarkably disappear.

Everything that happens to an unused muscle is bad—you're not only compromising your health, you're also not living up to your full potential as a human being. Not as much blood travels through an unused muscle, which means that muscle won't get enough oxygen and calcium, which means your tendons and ligaments become fragile. Eighty percent of all lower back pain may be due to muscular deficiency rather than pathology. Often, all you need to beat your back problems is a stronger back. And what's the only way to get a stronger back? That's right. Weight training. And women, listen to this. Studies show that you are more likely to develop osteoporosis than men; that's where your bones weaken and you start to hunch over as you get older. You already have less bone density than a man, and after menopause you lose even more bone density. One great solution is weight training.

And don't forget the great lesson you learned at the start of this book. The more lean muscle you have on your body, the more your metabolism rises. Conclusion? A weightlifting program is going to blast away your body fat. This won't happen during the actual training, but as a result of the training.

The Weight Program

Even in modest amounts, weight training is going to change you— as long as you know the right way to do it. I'm not saying that you must turn your living room into a weight room with big cast-iron dumbbells. In fact, I want you to throw away all your old conceptions about weight training, and give me a chance to re-inspire you.

I am not going to make a bodybuilder out of you. But I will steal a few pages from the bodybuilder's life-style. Whether you love them or hate them, they have attained a muscular development and low body-fat level that was unheard of years ago.

Let me stop right here, however, and say something to women. I know many of you are afraid to lift weights because you think you'll look like men. You don't want to get a huge body. You see women bodybuilders who have male-like muscles and you run screaming for your life. Relax. You're not going to come even close to such a program. The North Program is your quickest way to a more feminine body. I'm not putting you through two-a-day routines like women bodybuilders.

We are never going to "get huge" (a favorite bodybuilder's term), we're not going to build bulging muscles. To create the North Body, you don't get sore, you don't gain through pain, you don't lift weights until you literally can't get the bar over your head. In my system, more weight is not great. To me, pain means only one thing—you're hurting.

I admit, weight training is going to be the most complex aspect of your program, which is why it's often neglected. But I'm going to make it very easy for you. All I ask is that you be consistent, and focus on what you're doing. You're on your way to creating a shapely, defined body.

Home or Gym?

First question. Should you do this at your home or at the gym?

There are, of course, advantages and disadvantages to both places. The advantages of having a home gym is that it's open twenty-four hours a day, and you save a lot of excess time if you don't have to drive, but can walk down the hall into your own work-out room. You can roll right out of bed and do a workout. You have complete privacy.

The advantage of a gym (which can be a private health club, a recreational center, or even a high school weight room) is that you've got constant supervision and the best equipment. You can find a workout partner who will help you tremendously, and you'll be further motivated by simply being around other people trying to accomplish the same thing you are.

At Home

Can you develop a North Body at home? The answer is yes. But you need certain equipment. If you decide to go the home route, you're going to have to spend some money. It's going to be very difficult to do the North Program with just a couple of dumbbells. You're going to need a certain amount of equipment, the kind that you can later add on to as you gradually increase your weight. Technology is coming up with great new equipment. Just make sure you're buying it from a quality store and not from a television commercial.

Unless you've got money to burn, you do not need one of those home stack units. I've yet to see one I like for under $2,500; you'd get bored or outgrow the others fairly quickly. Some of the machines are so heavy you'd probably have to put them in the garage to keep from ruining a floor. Also you would break some chains and pulleys along the way, so add in maintenance costs.

For the initial North Body weight program, you can put together a home gym for no more than $500. If you look in the classified ad sections of newspapers, you'll always find used weights for sale from people who worked out a couple of times and then gave it all up (obviously, they didn't read my book).

You need to buy a bench that lies flat but can adjust to forty-five-degree and ninety-degree angles. You need to get a series of fixed dumbbells. You are looking at them costing about thirty to forty cents a pound. Don't get plastic weights or the kind of weights that screw on and off. You want something that feels solid in your hand. You also need a straight bar with various barbell plates to add to it. A woman will want to get the following:

1. A variety of dumbbells between three and twenty pounds.
2. A straight bar with two two-and-a-half-pound plates, two five-pound plates, and four ten-pound plates.
3. With a bench, the total cost should be less than $350.

A man will want to get the following:

1. Dumbbells that should range from ten pounds to forty pounds.
2. A straight bar with four five-pound plates, four ten-pound plates, two twenty-five pound plates, and if you want, two thirty-five or even forty-five pound plates, but no more.
3. With a bench, the total cost should be less than $500.

You should go to a gym before starting a home program just to get a chance to try out weights and see what size weights will be most comfortable for you. Absolutely do not start a program without getting at least a couple of supervised sessions at a gym from an experienced weight trainer who can see what you're doing wrong.

Furthermore, I want you, even if you have the best home gym possible, to go a public gym once every couple of months, at least to try out its equipment and see what helps your body improve. As you get highly advanced, you'll inevitably have to graduate from your home operation to a commercial gym.

At the Gym

What kind of gym to look for? Find a serious, well-equipped gym where people go to train and not to stand around. I also suggest finding a gym close to your work or home, so you don't have to let it inconvenience you. If you can't afford $20-$150 a month for a private club, then you need to go to the high school or community college or recreation center, or YMCA closest to you.

After a speech I gave in a small Texas town, I had some ladies come up and say, "Larry, our problem is that we don't have a gym to go to in this town." I said, "Do you have a high school?" They said yes, but it was full of students. "Well," I said, "go ask the coach about using it on weekends or nights." A few weeks later, I got a letter from one of those small-town ladies and learned that fifteen of them meet at the high school gym three times a week.

Some gyms are indeed expensive, but they usually have different membership rates throughout the year. The off-season in the gym world is late summer; you can get discounts up to 50 percent. Still, if you're looking at a really expensive gym, you need to ask yourself whether you'll be using expensive juice bars or saunas or massage rooms or the outdoor tennis courts that you'll be paying for.

When picking a gym, watch for these things:

1. While talking to a salesman, if you feel that you are on the witness stand being forced to give testimony about your body, walk out. They're trying to make you feel so guilty you're not in shape that you'll pay anything to join. Don't listen to high-pressure pitches.

2. Study the contract closely, looking for any hidden fees.

3. Visit the club at the time of day you plan to use it. It might be one thing to like a club when you're there on a lunch break, but if you're going to use it at 6:00 p.m., you need to see how crowded it is at that time.

4. Take your time looking the gym over. If the salesperson is rushing you, you need to wonder if something is wrong.

5. If you're going to change clothes at the gym, then spend time in the locker room. If you're going to feel uncomfortable or unclean taking a shower and dressing there, look for another club. Little things such as lack of comfort can amazingly keep you out of your own gym.

Do You Need a Trainer?

This book is designed to be your trainer. If you want to get a personal trainer, that's great, but expect to pay from $25 to $125 an hour. Make sure your trainer not only can supervise a weight program for you, but can lay out a nutrition plan, and motivate you; he or she should look like they practice what they preach.

Even with a personal trainer, you still need this book. Your first three to six weight sessions should be considered as mostly instructional lessons—not pure workouts. The huge mistake people make is that they go into their first weight day hoping to really train hard. But you should be there initially to learn. The first couple of workouts aren't going to make a massive difference in your physique. The next 120 workouts will. The number-one rule for weight training hasn't changed in one hundred years. The top professionals still follow it, and so should beginners.

Gym Talk

If you're going to be true to the North Program, you not only have to walk the walk, but talk the talk. You're about to learn a whole new language that is spoken in the weight room. If you don't pick up these terms, you'll never know what anyone is talking about:

Rep—An abbreviation of the word repetition (perhaps because muscle heads cannot pronounce "repetition"), a rep is the movement required to do a single weightlifting exercise.

Set—The number of repetitions performed on one exercise.

A spot—When someone stands behind you, watching you perform a set, making sure you finish your last rep so the bar won't land on your head and kill you.

"One More!"—A term that trainers or spotters use when they want you to perform three to five more repetitions.

Pumped—The feeling you get after a certain point in your workout that feels like all blood has been concentrated in your muscles, making them feel larger.

Burn—When you are at the end of a set, and the muscle you are exercising feels like it's on fire.

Flat—When your muscle can't get a pump no matter how hard you try.

Smooth—A person who has little or no definition in his muscles.

Defined—A person who has good muscularity.

Cut—A person who is extremely well-defined.

Ripped—A person who is so well cut that he looks like the model for an anatomy chart.

Shredded—Even more muscularity than ripped.

Body Parts

You also need to understand your body parts, all of which go by various silly abbreviations:

Bi's (pronounced: "Byes")—The biceps muscle in front of the arm. This is the infamous glory body part. When a guy makes a muscle to impress a girl, he's flexing his bi's.

Tri's (pronounced: "Tries")—The triceps muscle on the back of the arm. To make your bi's look good, you've got to work on your tri's.

Pecs—The chest muscles.

Lats—Your upper back muscles that give you that beautiful V-shape taper down to your waist.

Delts—Your deltoids, which are your shoulder muscles. They are often referred to by some women as "bumps."

Abs—Stomach muscles. What you someday hope to bounce a quarter off of.

Glutes—Your gluteus, or rear end, also known by some trainers (depending on their level of sophistication) as your buttocks, tushie, butt, bootie or glutes.

Quads—The front thigh muscle.

Hams—The hamstrings, or back of the leg muscles above the knees.

Calves—The back muscles in the lower leg. One of the most beloved muscles because they make your legs look great—but also one of the most difficult to develop.

Your Reps and Sets

Just so we all know we're on the same page here, I want to make sure you know that to properly complete a weight-training exercise that you will learn in the next chapter, you must do that exercise a certain number of times. If you remember the "Gym Talk" section, you must complete a certain number of reps for that exercise. Once you do those reps, you have completed a set. In the beginning, I'll never ask you to do more than ten reps in a row for each exercise. You take a break, and then you'll do another set of ten reps. Got it?

Some people will tell you to rest thirty seconds between sets; others say to rest sixty seconds between sets. I suggest you rest as long as you need to. Listen to your heart. I want you to never go so quickly that the strain takes away from the set that you are doing. Larger muscle groups and heavier exercises will require a little bit more rest than smaller muscle groups and lighter exercises.

When you train, here's what each set should do for you:

1. First Set—Choose a weight with which you can perform ten repetitions with perfect form. If you can do fifteen perfect reps, then you know you have picked too light a weight.

2. Second Set—You will be able to get in eight or nine perfect reps with perfect form, but that last rep will show a slighter flaw in your form. But that doesn't mean you yank, twist or cheat the weight to finish the second set.

3. Third Set—Try again for the same effect as the second set. You may have to drop a little bit of weight to get the eight or nine perfect reps before faltering again. You may add a tiny iota of body language to get the weight up for the tenth rep.

Form Is Everything

Technique determines whether you improve in weight training. The amount of weight is never the way to determine your success. You must never sacrifice form for weight. I'll be repeating this lesson over and over as I take you through specific weight training. Never sacrifice form so that you can finish an exercise.

The secret to insuring good form is posture. In life, you don't have to walk around as if you're a Marine standing at attention. But you do when you lift weights. You will rarely ever see a weight movement performed incorrectly with someone who has perfect posture. That means, in almost every exercise, your back is going to stay straight, your shoulders will be back, the chest will stick out, and the legs remain straight but not locked in position. If you find your shoulders slumping or your back rounding off or your hips thrusting forward or your back jerking to lift a barbell, then you are lifting incorrectly—and dangerously.

Good Posture

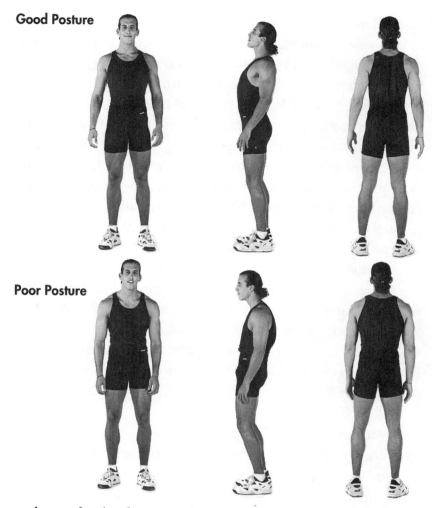

Poor Posture

As you begin, the pace of your reps is very important. Slow it down. Try for a rhythmic consistency. It's not necessary that you ever let a weight down faster or slower than you come up. Again, the key word to remember is control. You must control the weight. If you're losing control of the movement, you're doing it too fast. If you're going fast just to get the weight up, then you're using too much weight. After the first several reps of an exercise, you should feel the muscle you're working. If you don't, you're doing your reps too fast.

Lesson Two—Range of Movement

In your weight-training program, you always want to get the fullest range of motion that you can. How many people do you see in a weight room doing half movements with a lot of weight? You'll see them do the standard barbell curl about halfway up, then they go not all the way down. If they cut their weight in half and did a full motion, they'd see their muscles develop three times as fast.

You generally want to go all the way up and all the way down. With the exception of only a couple of movements with legs and certain back exercises (which we'll talk about later), you are trying to get a full extension when you drop the weight down and a full contraction when you lift it up. If you find yourself stopping midway through the movement, you're using too much weight.

Once and for all, get this through your head: Less is more. The only way to improve is to use less weight. Indeed, the amount of weight you use is almost insignificant, because if you do the exercise properly, you can take a light weight and make it feel heavy and get as much benefit out of it as using a heavier weight with sloppier form.

Keep Moving

You do not want to hold the weight at the top or the bottom of the movement. Keep constantly moving, which will keep constant tension in your muscles throughout a set of exercises. Don't ever rest the bar on your chest, or lock out and hold it for a couple of seconds at the top—that can lead to injury. Your weight-training program should be an eternal flow of motion, almost like rowing a boat where you never let the oars stop moving.

Breathing

This seems silly. Everyone breathes, right? Wrong. A lot of people hold their breath when they lift, which causes them to tense up and destroy their form and use muscles that don't need to be involved in a particular exercise. Get in the habit of being relaxed in the weight room. That means not to grip the bar so tightly that your knuckles turn white. That means you shouldn't grimace with your face or clench your teeth. And most importantly, that means to breathe naturally. The only muscle group that should be tense is the muscle that you're working on at the time.

It's important, in the beginning, to lift weights with your mouth open. As you get more advanced, you'll want to exhale as you exert the weight, and inhale as you let the weight down. But for now, just breathe. Make sure to inhale at the beginning of each movement.

Focus

In weight training, you have got to concentrate as if you were driving on a crowded highway. In the gym, I see too many people's minds wandering. You have got so many things to think about—posture, range of motion—that you should not have time to think about anything else. Learn to feel every exercise you perform. Learn to focus directly on the muscle part you're supposed to be working. Often, you'll hear an experienced weight lifter say, "Feel the movement" or "Feel the muscle." This takes time and concentration. But once you get there, you vastly improve.

Don't Get Sore

Once again, muscle soreness is not a sign of muscle progress. Safe and sane is what we're going for. Your sore muscles are not due to your completing an excellent workout. Your muscles don't get bigger because they get sore. I want you to get the right kind of feeling—a pulling sensation that stretches the muscle naturally.

Rest Your Body

Here's another one of those ironies that beginners cannot seem to understand: Your muscles won't get any stronger if you do not let them rest.

Anyone who tries to lift weights twice a day is doomed. You only have to lift weights at most three times a week. After being intensively exercised, a muscle needs about forty-eight hours—sometimes seventy-two hours—of rest to make its best progress. Overtraining can lead to injury, of course, but it also leads to a loss of muscle. That's right. You'll wear down the muscle so much it won't have the strength to grow.

You also don't need your weight workouts ever to last longer than sixty minutes; sometimes thirty minutes is all you need. The workouts need to be at a good comfortable pace, and you need to develop a nice rhythm as you move from one movement to another. But don't feel you have to spend a long time there.

Now, you're ready to hit the weight room. Just like your eating program, I want you to get in the habit of being very regular with your workouts for the first six weeks. Missing a couple of workouts isn't going to break your physique. But you're going to find your body will thrive on a regular workout, especially at the beginning. If you don't miss a workout, your body will develop more quickly.

Also, make sure you carry your workout diary. I would recommend that before you start each session, you write down the weight exercises you want to do and carry your diary with you the entire time you're in the weight room. Check off each routine as you finish it. Such a small gesture keeps you infinitely more focused.

Okay, get ready for your own body transformation.

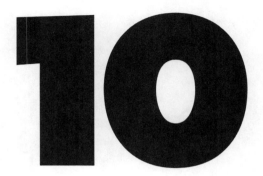

The Full-Body Weight Program
Exercises to
Resculpt Your Body

veryone is always asking me what the "ideal" exercise is for this body part or that body part. They are always trying to add a new kind of weightlifting movement to their reper- toire. They latch on to the latest new thing they see someone else do in a gym. They believe they have to do all these movements all the time to get the right body. I'm sorry, but there is no secret exercise. There is no one "Ideal Weight Training Movement of All Time." Basically, we are doing the same movements we've done since weightlifting began. Yes, there are lots of routines, and at some point you should listen to various experts. But for now, I want you to learn the ones that are the easiest to complete and over the years have provided the best results for muscles.

First, I'm going to give you two basic exercises for each major body part—which are the same exercises that the most advanced bodybuilders use, regardless of how many other exercises they know. Then, I'm going to give an additional exercise for those of you who work out at a gym and have access to certain machines. Finally, I'm going to give a fourth exercise for those who are at the level of advanced training.

Your routine might seem simple—but again, I want to tell you, you do not need to worry about all the other weight-training exercises you might see being done in gyms. Many beginning weightlifters disastrously miss out on the fundamental weightlifting routines, which is why it takes so long for their bodies to graduate to intermediate or advanced levels. This program hits every muscle group and will remain your foundation forever.

Beginners: Go Slowly

Please, for any of you who've been out of the gym for a while or who have never been there, do one thing for me. Go slowly. Do not try to lift very much in your first weeks. If you get yourself sore—and you won't if you follow my instructions—then you'll lie in bed the next morning, hardly able to move your body, cursing me and the North Program. You won't come back to the weight room, and you'll ultimately let a golden opportunity pass you by. So, for the beginners, here's what you should do to ease into the weight program:

First Week—You should perform only one exercise for each of the body parts that I discuss here. That means one chest exercise, one back exercise, and so on. Do only one set, lasting ten reps, using a weight that does not require any strain whatsoever. Worry about form only, not weight. Your first few weight workouts should last maybe fifteen to twenty minutes each. If at the end of the first week, you're saying this is all too easy, then you're doing everything perfectly.

Second Week—You're going to keep doing only one exercise per body part. But now move up to two sets per exercise for the major muscle groups, while remaining with one set for the smaller muscle groups. Continue to avoid any strain whatsoever. If you're starting to think I'm really too easy—if you're saying, "Come on, Larry, let me at these weights"—then you are still on the perfect pace.

Third Week—You're going to gradually pick up your pace. You will do two exercises, two sets each, on your major muscle groups.

And you'll do one exercise, two sets each, on your minor muscle groups. Pick and choose weights you are comfortable and confident with. Absolutely no straining! By the end of the third week, try for the regular routine.

The Regular Routine

When you are ready for the regular routine, all you have to do is:

1. Pick out two exercises for each larger muscle group category. Two exercises for the chest, two for the back, two for the shoulders, two for the glutes and two for the quads. On each exercise, you'll do two to three sets of ten reps each.

2. Pick out one exercise for each smaller muscle group. On each exercise, you'll do two to three sets of biceps, triceps, hamstrings and calves.

3. Keep each session no longer than forty to sixty minutes. You should do your weight routines two to three times a week for the next six to eight weeks. Nothing more. Don't think that because two sets felt good, then obviously five sets would make you feel better. That's a classic mistake. Once you've learned the exercises, and your body has acquired some stamina, then your goal should be to do three perfect sets—but no more. You do not want to overdo your muscles.

If I have to say this a thousand times, I will. A weight workout is never meant to wear you out. You don't want to feel completely drained. You never want to feel like you can't move a muscle. You want to feel exhilarated, not exhausted. On those days you don't feel up to par or feel a little fatigued, don't miss a workout—just perform all of your sets at a lighter level, where you can get in ten reps with perfect form and not worry about straining. You'll still be amazed at how much your muscles respond.

(NOTE: Be aware that the last photo in each exercise sequence—unless otherwise captioned—depicts the INCORRECT way of performing the exercise. Directions accompanying these "incorrect" photos reinforce proper weight-training techniques.)

The Weight Exercises

Chest:

Let's start with the ultimate glory body part. Men see a strongly developed chest as the ultimate symbol of masculine strength. Women think of stronger pecs as their chance to get bigger breasts. Actually, chest exercises won't change the size of the mammary glands, but they will keep the breasts from sagging. By strengthening your pectoral muscles, you'll make your breasts firmer simply by giving them a muscular foundation.

CHEST: Incline Press.

The incline press is better on your back and will help develop the usually neglected upper chest better than the traditional flat bench press. In the traditional bench press, men tend to use too much weight and end up straining too hard.

- Using either a barbell or dumbbells, lie with your back flat on a forty-five-degree-angle bench. Elbows should stick out parallel from your shoulders.

Jean Robert Barbette

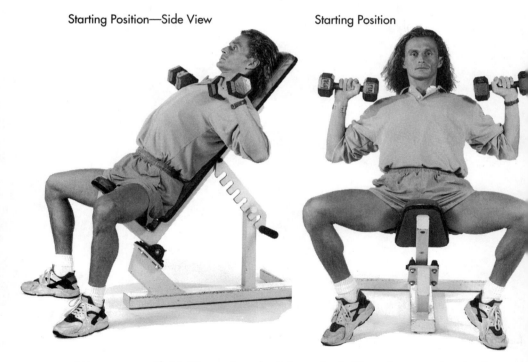

Starting Position—Side View   Starting Position

Women, start with 15-20 pounds total weight on a barbell (warning: a regular-sized barbell will weigh 15-20 pounds, so you don't need to add extra weight). If you are using dumbbells, start with eight pounds for each dumbbell. Men, start with 45-65 pounds total weight on a barbell or use fifteen-to-twenty-pound dumbbells.

- Push up and back, almost in an arc over your head. Most people make a mistake in pushing too far out in front of them. If you go out instead of straight up, you'll work more of your shoulder than your chest. It's important to stretch fully at the bottom of the movement and to flex the chest as you push up.

- If you use dumbbells, push up with your palms facing forward, and be sure to push in a triangular motion, so that the dumbbells come up like a pyramid. At the top, the dumbbells should come close together, but never touch.

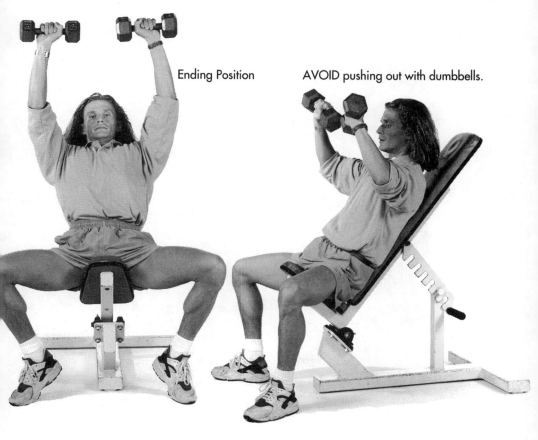

Ending Position

AVOID pushing out with dumbbells.

CHEST: Flat Bench Flies.

This is not like a "press" in which you take the weights up and down. Here, we're going to fly.

- Take a dumbbell in each hand and extend the arms fully above you while you're lying on a flat bench. As you go down, keep the arms straight, but definitely not locked out; keep a slight bend in the elbow. You only want to bring the weight down so the arms are parallel to the ground.

Jack Heizelman

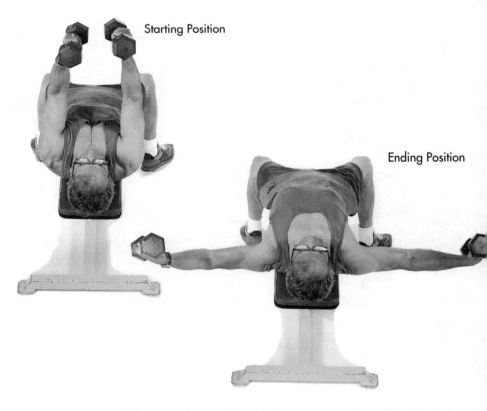

Starting Position

Ending Position

Women, start with five- to eight-pound dumbbells. Men, use twelve- to fifteen-pound dumbbells.

- Then go back up, bringing the weights to a point about three to five inches from each other. You need to pretend you have a barrel on your chest and that you are trying to bring the dumbbells around the outside of the barrel.

- You want the weights to be above your chest when you're at the top of the movement and then parallel with your shoulders at the bottom of the movement. Note: you can do this exercise on a forty-five-degree incline bench to work your upper chest. You can also do it on a decline bench to work your lower chest.

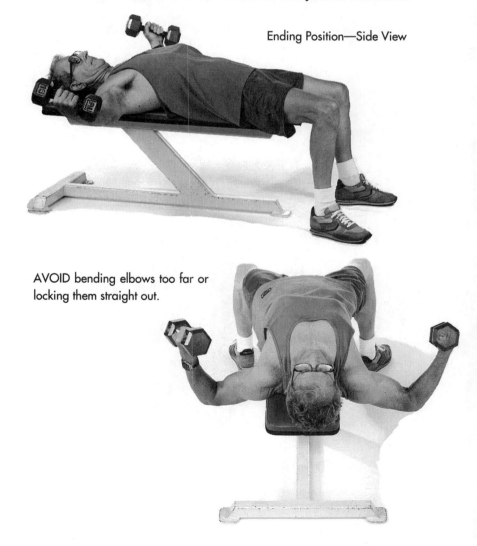

Ending Position—Side View

AVOID bending elbows too far or locking them straight out.

CHEST [Gym]: The Pec Deck
(also known as the butterfly.)

- Sit in the chair of the machine and adjust the seat so that a straight line can be drawn between the bottom part of your elbow and the lower part of your shoulder.

Adam North

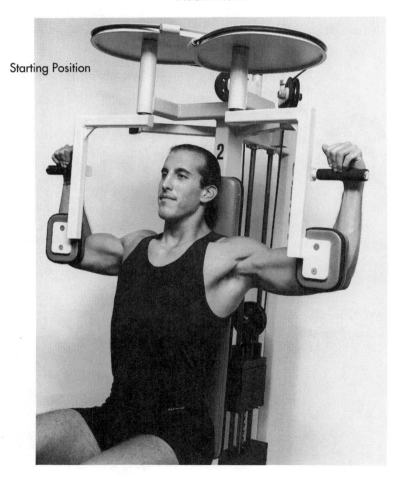

Starting Position

- Let the weight stretch your arms back to where the chest feels stretched, then slowly bring the weight forward, squeezing and flexing the chest the entire time.

Ending Position

AVOID adjusting seat too high, thus making elbows too low and head too far forward.

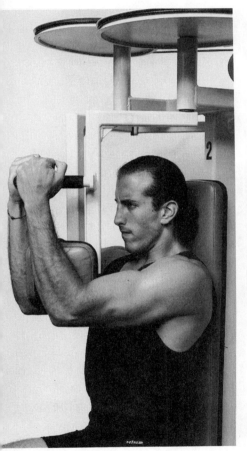

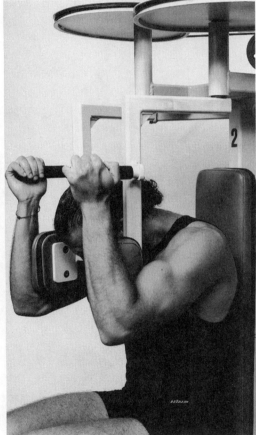

CHEST: Advanced Dips

One of the great exercises for the chest. This can be done at the gym or at home (a handyman can easily install some parallel bars in your home).

Starting Position   Ending Position

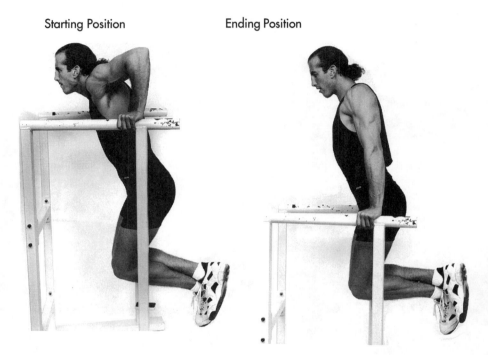

- When doing dips to build the chest, you generally want the elbows out, not in. Put your hands on the bars beside your body. Then dip down, deep enough to get a good stretch in the chest.

- When you come up, don't lock out with your arms fully straight. Come up about three-quarters of the way. Always keep focused on the chest muscle, trying to keep it tense.

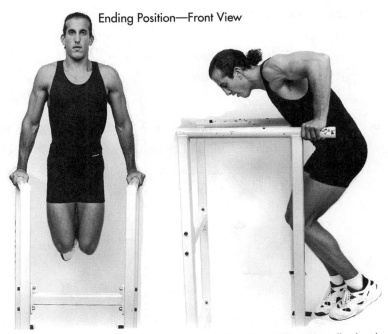

Ending Position—Front View

Keep the back straight and really dip down.

Back

The back gets neglected as much as any body part, mainly because you can't see it. So you have to especially concentrate on your back, because you have an array of different muscles in your upper back, middle back and lower back. If you have undeveloped back muscles, your shoulder blades will stick out like big bony knobs. An undeveloped upper back will also make the waist look too big and wide. Ideally, you want your upper body to taper into a tight V as it comes to your waist—and to do that, you've got to build your back.

In each of the following exercises, you have to pay a lot of attention to keeping your back straight. You'll hurt your lower back if you are working out in a bent-over position. Also, make sure not to grip the bar of your weight too tightly in these exercises, or else you'll make the arm muscles do a lot of the work. If you lighten up on your grip and practice stretching the back in between each set, it will help you learn to feel the back muscles doing the work.

BACK: One-Arm Dumbbell Rows

- Put your left knee on a flat bench and keep your right foot on the floor. With the dumbbell in the right hand, lean over and put your freed-up left hand on the front part of the bench to support yourself.

- With the weight dropped all the way down, rotate your shoulder upward as you lift the dumbbell to your waist. Then slowly bring the weight down, feeling the back muscles stretch until your arm is fully extended.

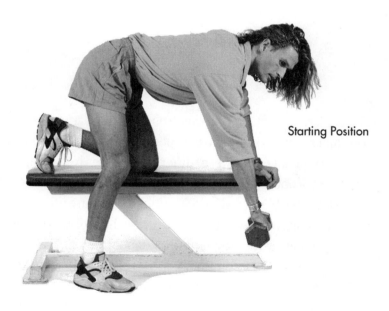

Starting Position

Women, begin with ten-pound dumbbells. Men, use twenty- to twenty-five-pound dumbbells.

- But don't let the weight go straight down. Bring the weight down at an angle so it ends up at the front of the body. Then repeat the movement by switching legs and switching the weight to the hand on the other side.

- Always, in this exercise, keep the back slightly arched. And never jerk the weight up when doing the one-arm row, or you'll hurt your lower back. If you feel a need to jerk, stop the exercise immediately and get a lighter weight.

Keep your back slightly arched and your elbows close to the body.

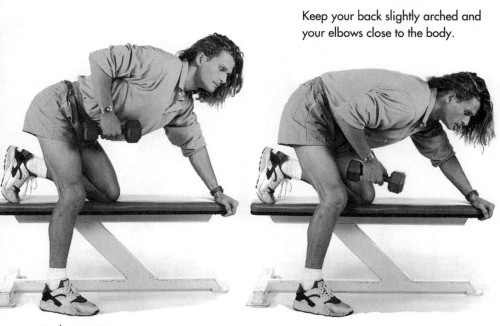

Ending Position

BACK: Bent-Over Row.

This is like the exercise you just learned, only it involves two arms and a barbell.

- Your knees must always remain slightly bent. Bend over until your back becomes parallel with the ground. Bend your knees to pick up the bar, and keep your grip shoulder-width apart. You can use an overhand grip or underhand grip.

Starting Position—Front View　　Starting Position—Side View

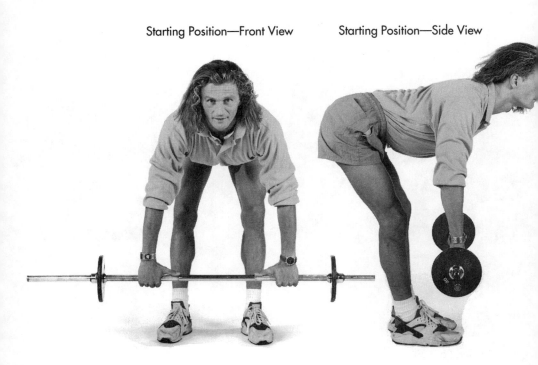

Both men and women, start this exercise using only the bar without weight until you feel comfortable putting weight on.

- Keep your shoulders straight, chest out, and now pull the bar to the lower chest or to the upper stomach. Then slowly go down so that the arms are fully extended.

- As you pull back upward, you do want to pull the shoulders back, almost as if you are trying to make the back of your shoulder blades touch one another. It's harder to breathe in this position, which makes it important to concentrate on your breathing.

Ending Position

AVOID bending or bowing your back and shoulders.

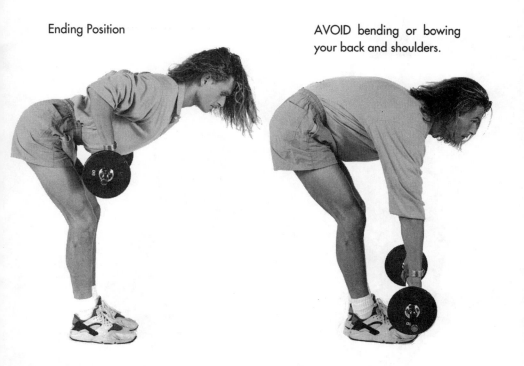

BACK [Gym]: Lat Pull-downs.

- Using a close-together grip or a wide grip, grab the bar above you and pull down to the top of the chest or the bottom of the chin. Pulling any lower works the shoulders more than it works the back. In the past, a lot of people were taught to pull behind the head; actually, pulling behind the neck puts undue stress on your neck and the lower back.

Alan North

Starting Position   Ending Position

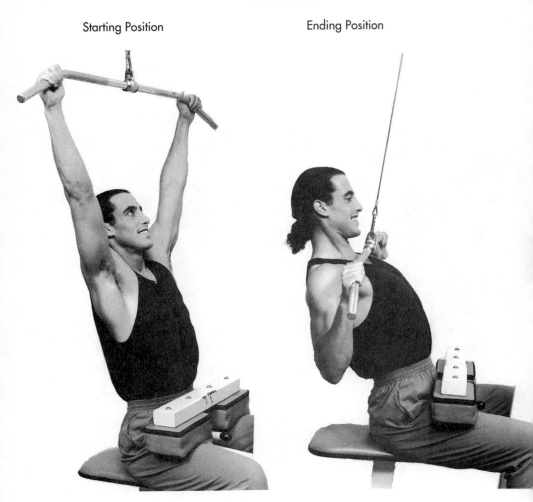

- The key to lat pull-downs is the extension. As you pull down, allow your back to lean back very slightly. Then as you go up with the weight, extend the arms until they are straight. As you do so, allow the torso to completely straighten out.

AVOID leaning back too far. Keep your shoulders back, and back straight.

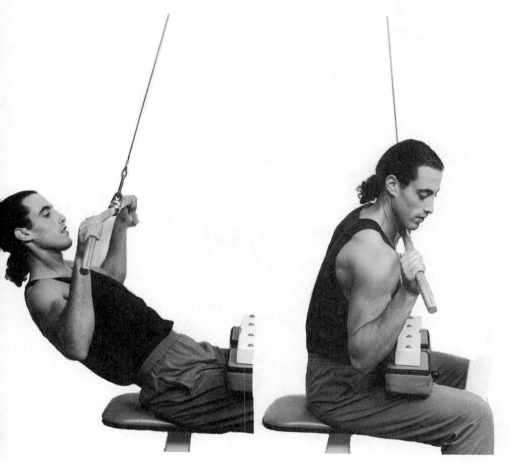

BACK: Advanced Pull-ups

The old-fashioned pull-up. Pull-ups and dips alone can build a nice upper body. For those strong enough to do pull-ups, there is no better exercise to get that V shape.

- Using either a close grip or wide grip, grab a chin-up bar (you can find one at any playground if you're not at a gym), pull your chest to the front of the bar, go down, and go back up for as many repetitions as you can.

Starting Position

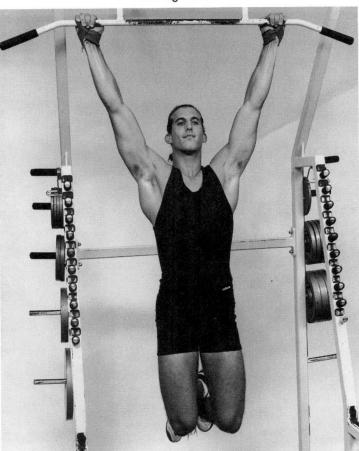

For those of you who are overweight, I would prefer you avoid this movement. And for those of you just beginning to do pull-ups, it's helpful to get a spotter. If you get stuck pulling yourself up, the spotter standing behind you can push up your knees.

Ending Position

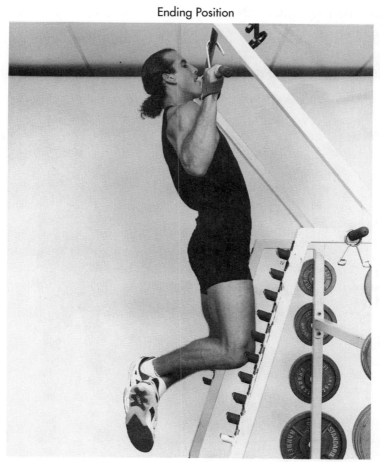

AVOID swinging during pull-ups. Also, AVOID this exercise if you've just begun a weight-training program.

Shoulders

There's no hiding poorly developed shoulders. They are one of the keys to good posture. They give width to the upper body (which can make your waist look smaller). Since your shoulders comprise a very small muscle group and gets worked in every single upper-body exercise you do, you don't require a lot of weight for these exercises. It's an easy muscle group to overtrain and injure. So you certainly should not work shoulders heavily. If you have a shoulder injury, or shoulder problem—which can mean any type of pain around the shoulder—then you might be best off not training the shoulder.

SHOULDERS: Upright Row.

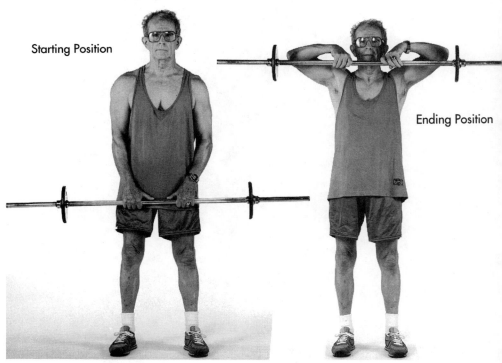

Starting Position

Ending Position

For women, start off with a fifteen-pound bar, and men start at thirty to forty pounds.

- With your hands six to eight inches apart as they hold the barbell (you can also use dumbbells), stand straight up, with your back perfectly straight and your feet a little narrower than shoulder width. Legs are slightly bent.

- With arms starting off extended straight down, pull the bar to the chin. Keep the knuckles of your hands pointed down at the ground for the entire movement, and keep the bar as close to your body as possible.

- Also keep your elbows higher than the bar through the movement. Let the bar down so you can get complete stretch at the bottom. Repeat.

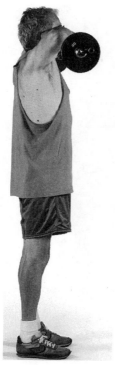

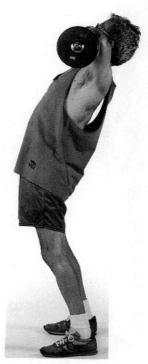

Ending Position—Side View

AVOID leaning too far back. Keep your back perfectly straight, your hands at least six inches apart, and your elbows higher than the barbell.

SHOULDERS: Side Lateral Raises.

- Using dumbbells, you can stand or remain seated on a bench or chair. Let your hands drop all the way down to the sides.

- Now send the arms and dumbbells straight out. Try to keep the arms straight, without locking out. The hands should always be in line with the shoulders.

Reggie Senegal

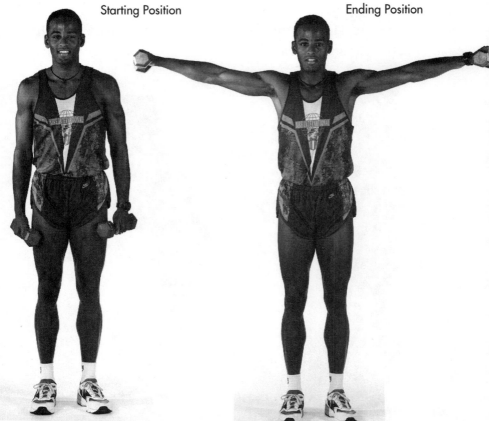

Starting Position   Ending Position

Women, use three- to five-pound dumbbells. Men should start with eight- to ten-pound dumbbells.

- The dumbbells should barely go higher than shoulder level, and then let them down slowly. Think of performing this movement the way a ballet dancer does that movement where she sends her hands flowing outward.

Move your arms out straight and smoothly, not forward and jerky. AVOID using too much weight.

Ending Position—Side View

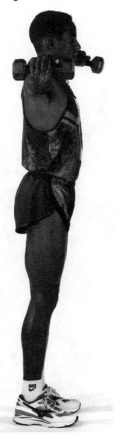

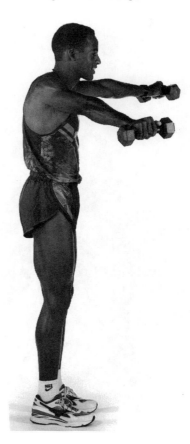

SHOULDERS [Gym]: Overhead Press.

Using either a machine, dumbbells or barbells, it's preferable to do this exercise seated because it puts less stress on the back.

- Hold the bar (or dumbbell) at shoulder width. Push straight up overhead, but don't push behind your head. Come down, and repeat.

Again a word of caution: Do not go heavy, and do not lift if you are fatigued. It's just not necessary.

Starting Position   Ending Position

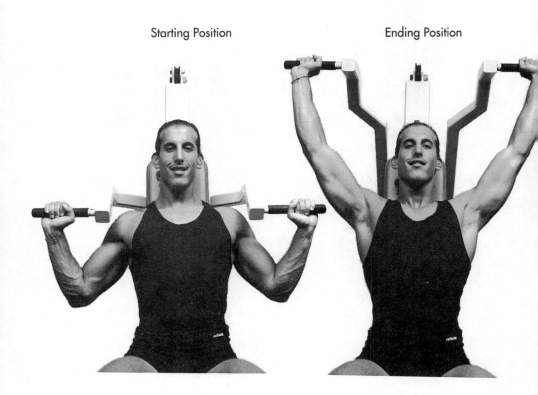

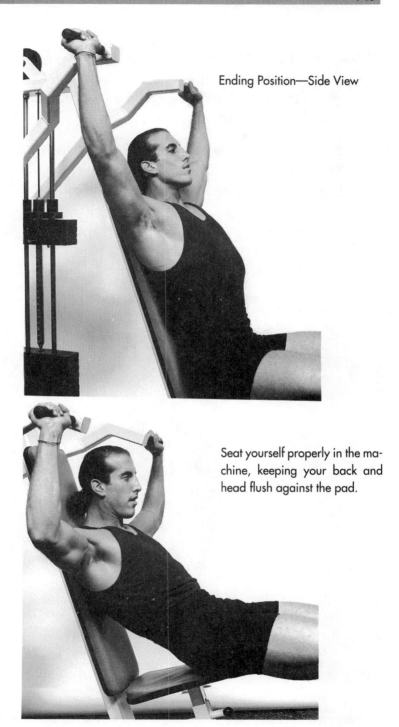

Ending Position—Side View

Seat yourself properly in the machine, keeping your back and head flush against the pad.

SHOULDERS [Advanced]: Bent-Over Lateral Raises.

- This exercise, working the rear part of the shoulders, requires that you sit on the edge of a chair or bench with a dumbbell in each hand.

- Bring your chest down to your thighs in a bent-over position. Then pull the dumbbell straight out, up to shoulder level. Keep the weights just slightly behind the body.

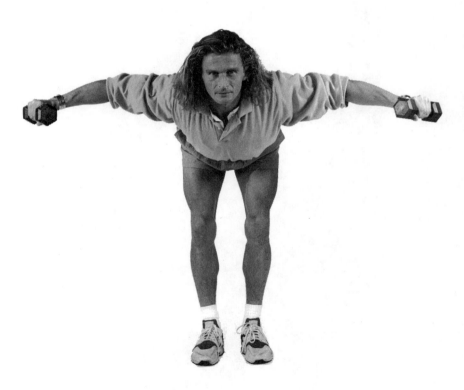

Women, start with three- to five-pound dumbbells. Men, use eight-pound dumbbells.

Keep your back straight and your arms out, and keep shoulders and elbows level.

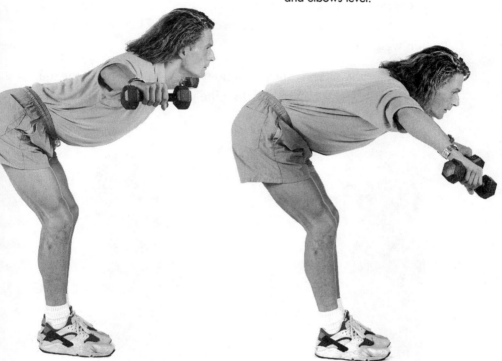

Glutes and Quads

The big leg muscles are usually neglected. For people training at home, there is little equipment to help them train their legs. Most men are usually so concerned with their upper body that they have a tendency to blow off leg workouts. Women tend to ignore leg training for fear they will develop big legs.

But the way to get legs shapely is through this training. Moreover, one thing you can especially develop through glute and quad work is a tight, round bottom, with minimal body fat and no cellulite. As an added benefit, leg training speeds up metabolism because the quads and glutes take up so much muscle mass in the body.

GLUTES AND QUADS: Larry Lunges

If all you did for your lower body was lunges, then you'd develop great legs. You can do lunges with dumbbells in your hand or with a bar on your shoulders or with no weight at all. They never require much weight.

- Beginners should start with no weight. Stand with your feet shoulder-width apart and imagine you are on railroad tracks.

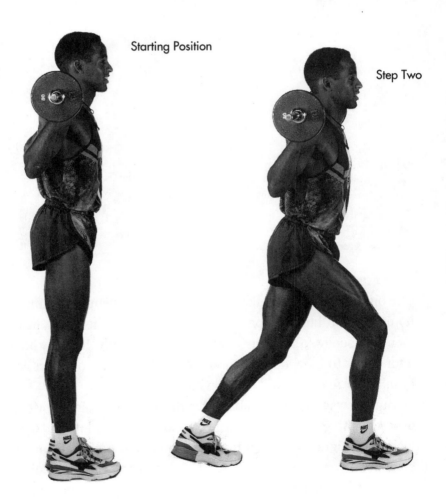

Starting Position

Step Two

- Take one foot and step forward as if you're taking one giant step forward in the old Simon Says game. When you step forward, your foot should go straight forward, like you're walking on a railroad track.

- As you step forward, bend your back leg, but never let the knee touch the ground. Then step back and alternate legs.

- If you want to put more emphasis on the muscles in your butt when stepping back, lift the toes of your front foot upward and push back on your heel. If you currently have knee problems, you might want to omit this exercise.

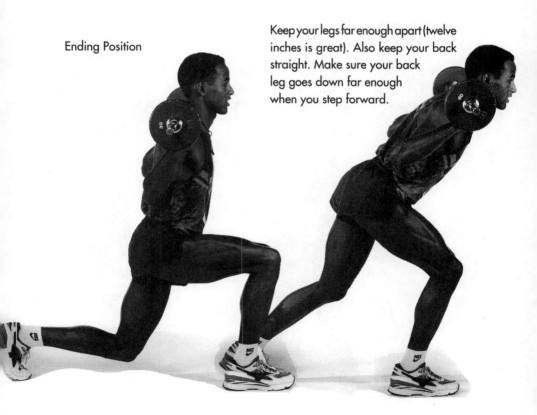

Ending Position

Keep your legs far enough apart (twelve inches is great). Also keep your back straight. Make sure your back leg goes down far enough when you step forward.

GLUTES AND QUADS: Front Squats

You do not need weight to learn this exercise; you do not even need to use a bar. This is a different kind of squat than what you've seen, because you are going to be putting the bar at the top of your chest, not behind your head on your shoulders.

- Just hold the bar as if you are going to do an overhead press. The reason you do this in front is to keep your back straight; it insures proper form and prevents injury.

Renee Redden

Starting Position—Front View   Starting Position

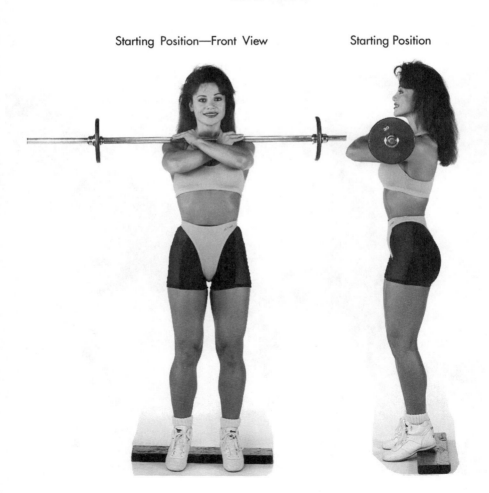

- Stand with your feet shoulder-width apart (For those of you who are beginners and don't have good flexibility, prop your heels up on a two-by-four.)

- Then simply pretend you're sitting down. Never let your butt go lower than your knees. When your thighs are parallel to the ground, lift back up—but don't lock out the knees at the top of the movement. Keep them slightly bent.

- If your knees bend towards one another and touch during this exercise, you're using too much weight. You do more reps than usual in this exercise, because you don't need much weight.

- Always keep your hands close to center of bar, with the elbows high—and make sure the bar is firmly in place at the top of the chest.

Ending Position

AVOID using so much weight that your thighs go past parallel and your knees touch.

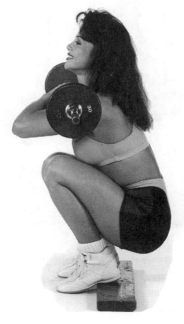

GLUTES AND QUADS [Gym]: Leg Extensions.

This is a big-time leg shaper, and you can do it without using heavy weight. You want to precisely control the movement. If you use too much weight, you'll start swinging the weight and lose control.

- Sit in the leg-extension machine and put your feet behind the pad. You want the pad to hit you right above the foot at the bottom of the ankle, so adjust it accordingly.

Starting Position   Ending Position

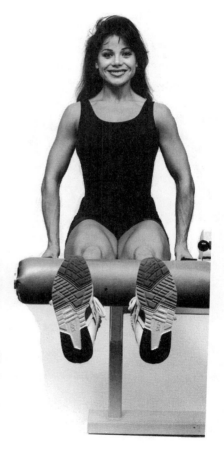

- Come up all the way with your legs, but don't come all the way back because it will put too much stress on the knees. Remember: Safety first. Go back down three-quarters of the way.

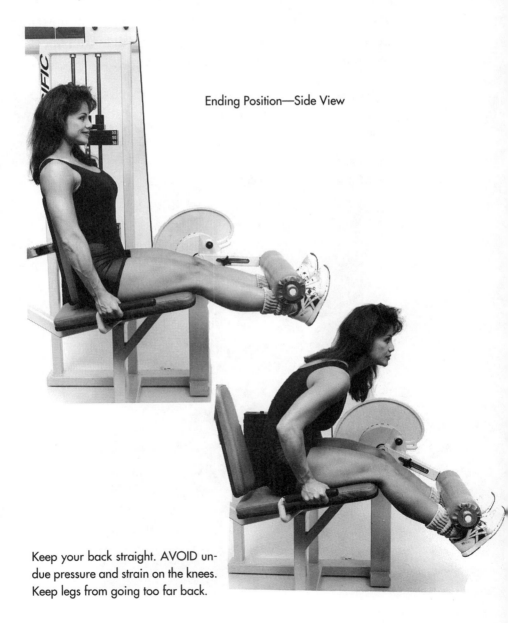

Ending Position—Side View

Keep your back straight. AVOID undue pressure and strain on the knees. Keep legs from going too far back.

GLUTES AND QUADS [Advanced]: Leg Press.

This is another machine, a forty-five-degree-angle leg press, that can work the thighs and the hips in a way you would not believe.

- Seated in the angled chair, put your feet on the platform. (The higher your heels are on the platform, the more butt muscle you'll work.) Always keep your heels higher than your knees, so as not to put too much stress on the knees.

- Push up on the platform, and never, never lock out your legs. Come down about three-quarters of the way, not all the way back.

Starting Position

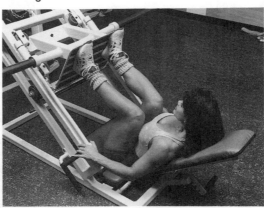

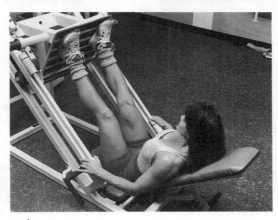

Ending Position

- The minute your butt starts to rise up off the seat, you're using too much weight or you're coming back too far and putting too much stress on the lower back.

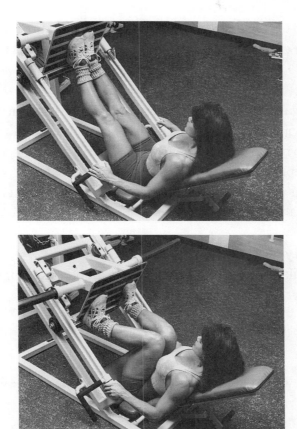

AVOID locking your knees (top photo). AVOID positioning knees higher than your feet. AVOID allowing the knees to touch, because stress belongs on the quads and glutes (bottom photo).

Smaller Muscle Groups

The smaller muscle groups automatically get worked as you train the larger muscles. And because there is not as much muscle there, you don't have to train them as hard. Still, I see guys doing tons of biceps exercises—when the fact is they are harming the muscle more than helping it.

For each smaller muscle, I'm only giving you three exercises— one exercise for everyone, then one gym exercise, and then one advanced exercise. If you're a beginner, you need to do only one of the three exercises.

Triceps

The tri's take up two-thirds of your upper arm, so when you think of developing great arms, you need to concentrate as much on tri's as you do bi's. When fully developed, the tri's make the upper arm look complete. It makes great sense to keep the tri's as toned and defined as possible so that you will not be subjected, later in life, to the old flabby arm problem.

TRICEPS: Lying Triceps Extensions.

- While lying flat on a bench, grab a barbell six to eight inches apart. Hold it straight above you.

Starting Position

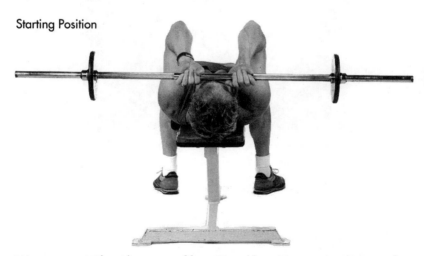

Women, start only with a ten- to fifteen-pound bar. Men, start with twenty-five to thirty pounds.

- Now, while keeping the elbows close together (you'll have to force your elbows inward because they'll want to veer out), bring the bar slowly down to the top of the forehead.

- Then push straight back up, where the bar ends up right above your head, not above your chest. You'll want your elbows to point straight toward the ceiling throughout the entire movement; the only parts of the arms that move are the forearms and wrists.

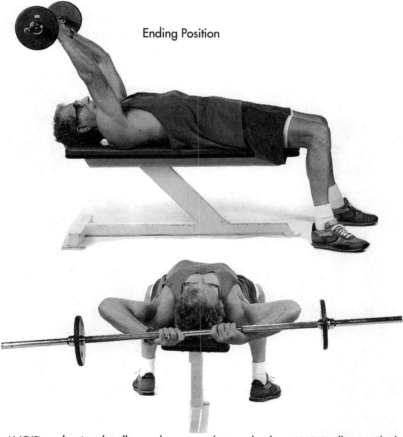

Ending Position

AVOID not having the elbows close enough to each other. AVOID allowing the bar to go behind the head. Try to keep your elbows parallel and aim the barbell toward your forehead.

TRICEPS [Gym]: Push-downs.

These are generally performed on a cable machine with a V-shaped bar (or a straight bar).

- Standing upright, with back straight and knees soft, lean slightly forward into the movement. Your elbows must remain in front of the body, not in back of the body or the sides of the body. This will ensure that you isolate the triceps.

Starting Position   Ending Position

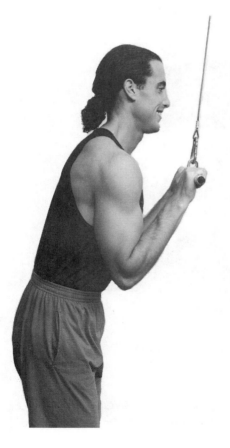 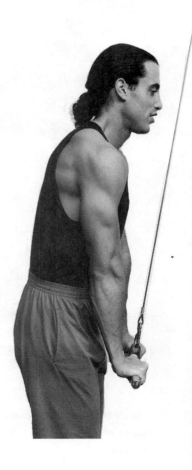

- Push downward, keeping your forearms parallel with one another, and get as full an extension as possible, just short of locking out.

Keep your arms in. Also, keep your elbows pointed outward.

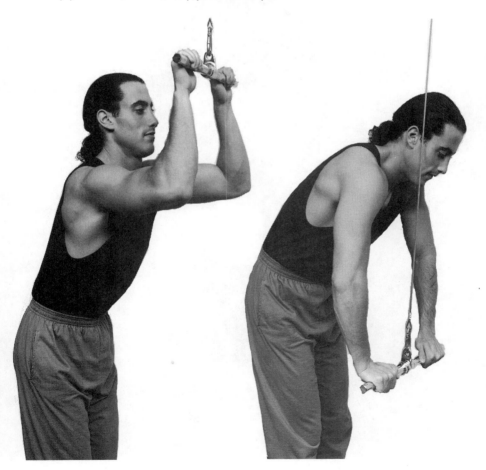

TRICEPS [Advanced]: Close-Grip Bench Press.

This is very similar to the lying tricep extension—except you're going to use more weight because you will push the bar straight up, just like your basic bench press. What's also different is that you keep your grip closer, just six to eight inches apart.

- Start with the bar at the bottom of the chest and push straight up, keeping the bar over your chest at all times.

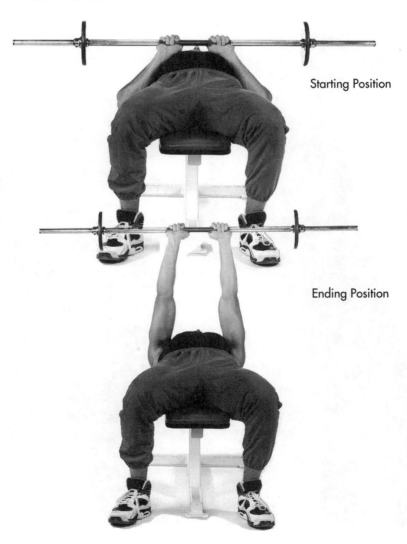

Starting Position

Ending Position

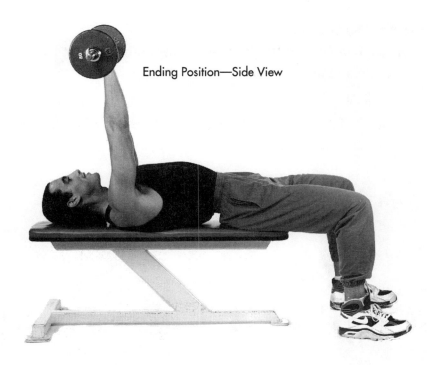

Ending Position—Side View

Women, start with fifteen pounds, men with forty-five to fifty-five pounds. Bring the bar to the middle of or the lower part of the chest, not the upper part of the chest.

Biceps

I think it's great that the nicely shaped biceps have become so important and sexy to a woman. For a man, of course, this is the other glory body part. But remember, the most common mistake you make doing biceps exercises is to overdo it. You're so desperate to get good biceps that you do too many sets or use too much weight.

BICEPS: The Straight-Bar Curl.

The all-time favorite weight exercise. Grab the straight bar narrower than shoulder width.

- Keeping the arms slightly in front of the body, pull up toward the chin, flex at the top, and then let the bar all the way down to the thighs.

Starting Position—Side View   Starting Position—Front View

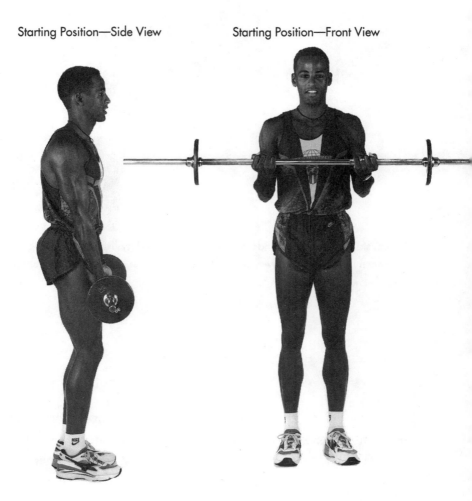

Women, start with fifteen pounds, men with thirty to forty pounds.

- The arms must remain parallel with one another, and your elbows should come up only a few inches as you get to the top of the movement.

- Good tip: When you start the movement from the bottom, pretend you're making a muscle for someone—and that will move the bar upward.

Ending Position

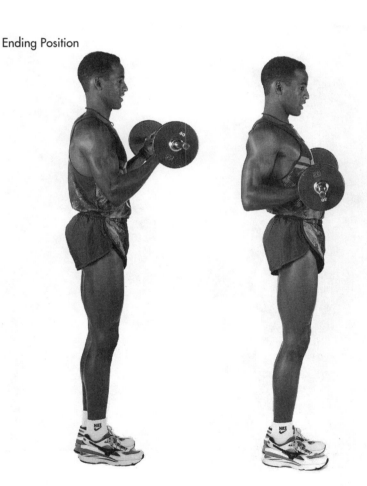

Keep your back straight, elbows forward, and legs slightly bent. AVOID swinging or jerking the bar up to the chin.

BICEPS [Gym]: Preacher Curls.

- Using either a straight bar, bent bar, or dumbbells, sit on the preacher bench and make sure the back of the arm always rests against the pad. You don't want to be seated so low that your armpits are touching the pad. You want about two inches space from the pad to your shoulder.

Starting Position   Starting Position—Side View

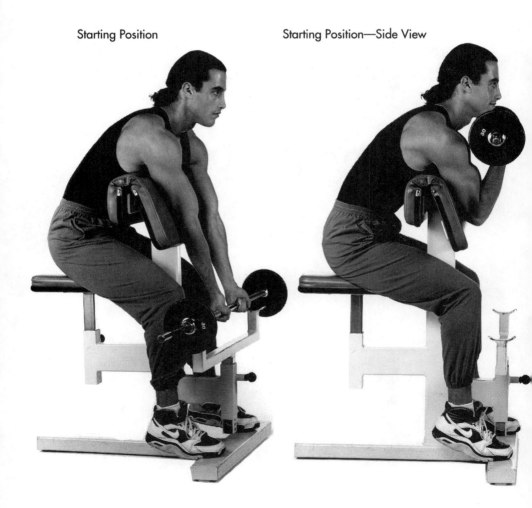

Women, use a bar with no added weight. Men, twenty-five to thirty pounds.

- With the elbows as close together as possible, the hands should grab the bar slightly wider than the elbows. Squeeze all the way up, then let the bar down about three-quarters of the way. Don't go all the way down because it puts too much pressure on your elbows and tendons.

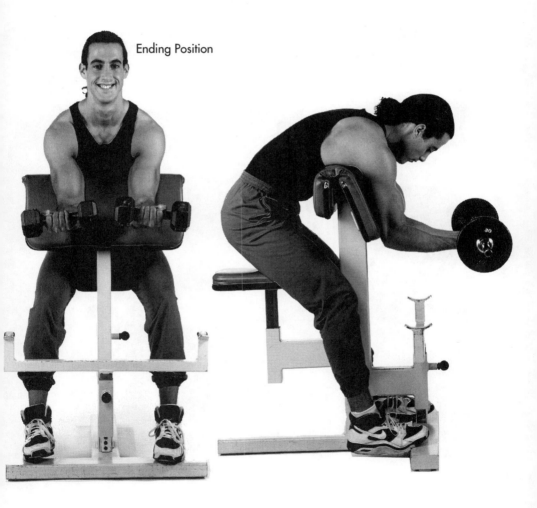

Ending Position

Keep about two inches of space between the armpit and the pad. Also, keep your butt down and your head up.

BICEPS [Advanced]: Incline Dumbbell Curls.

- Sitting on a forty-five-degree incline bench, put a dumbbell in each hand, and let your arms drop straight down so that your hands are directly below your shoulders.

- With your palms facing away from your body, raise the dumbbells up, making sure the pinkies of your hands are higher than your thumbs (this will isolate the biceps). You don't need to use heavy weights here.

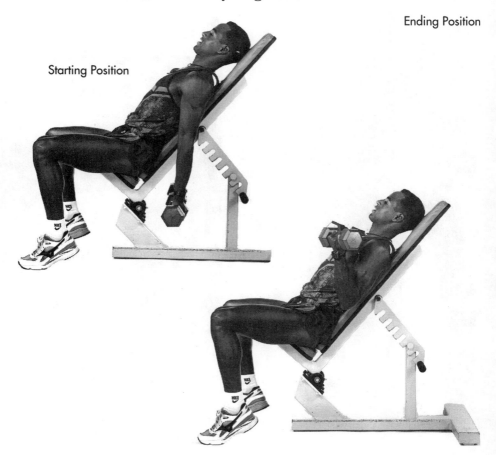

Ending Position

Starting Position

Women, start with five-pound dumbbells. Men, start with twelve-pound dumbbells.

Ending Position—Front View

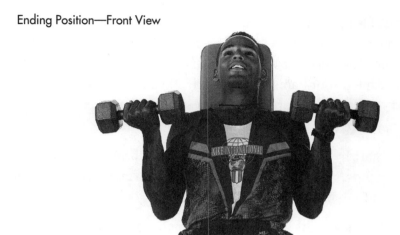

Keep your elbows in, your pinkies higher than your thumbs, and the dumbbells even.

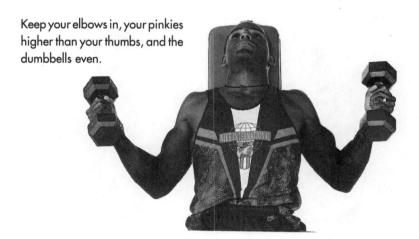

Hams

The hamstrings are highly neglected, and yet they are one of the keys to developing a nice rear end. Few things on the body are more attractive than developed hamstrings. When worked properly, your hams look like long muscles on a beautiful race horse. Regardless how developed the rest of your lower body is, without having adequate hamstrings the lower body looks incomplete.

HAMS: Straight-Leg Deadlifts

Because there are so few exercises for the hams, I'm giving you an advanced exercise. Be very careful. If you do this correctly, nothing can develop your hams more quickly. If you do it wrong, you can hurt your lower back. (If you feel any strain in the lower back at any time, you're doing this movement wrong.)

- Start by holding just a bar (or even a broomstick) in your hands, shoulder-width apart, with your arms dropped directly in front of you down by your thighs.

- Now lower the bar to four to five inches below the knees (less

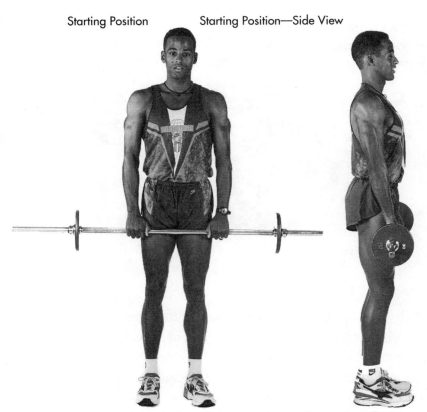

Starting Position   Starting Position—Side View

Women and men both need to start with just a bar and no weight.

if you aren't flexible enough to go down that far). Try to feel the stretch in your hamstrings.

- As you lower the bar, you want your buttocks to push out in the opposite direction. Despite its name, this movement is not performed with straight legs; do not lock out your knees.

- Keep your shoulders back and chest out the entire time, and don't let your shoulders come forward as you bend forward. Once you feel a slight stretch in the hamstring, just slowly straighten yourself up.

Ending Position

AVOID a rounded back, locked-out legs and letting the bar fall too far below the knees.

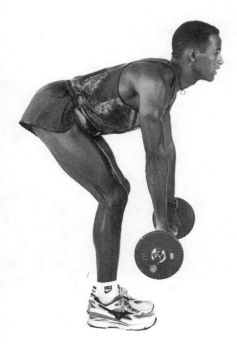

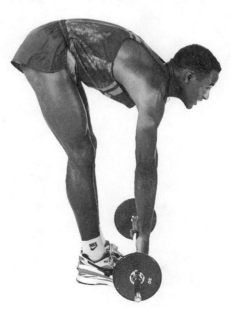

HAMS [Gym]: Lying Down Leg Curls

- Lie flat on the leg curl bench. Adjust the foot pad so it hits two inches above your heel. Relax the foot at all times.

- Lift up the pad, making sure you come all the way up until the pad hits your hamstrings, then come only three-quarters of

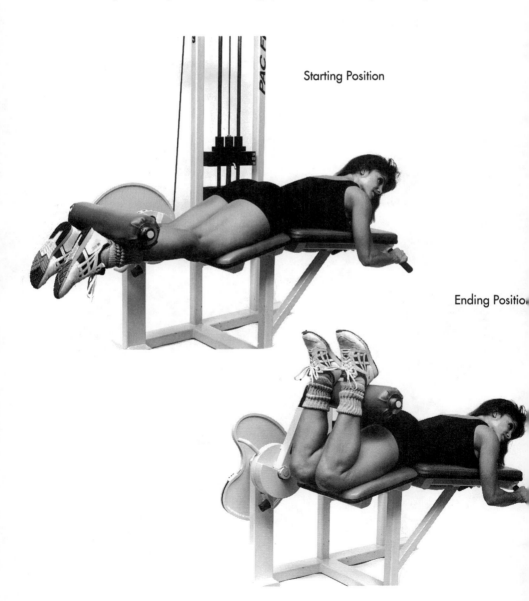

Starting Position

Ending Position

the way down. You want to limit your range of motion here in your legs, because you don't want additional stress in the lower back.

- The most common mistake made in this exercise is to use too much weight, which causes the hips to rotate in the air.

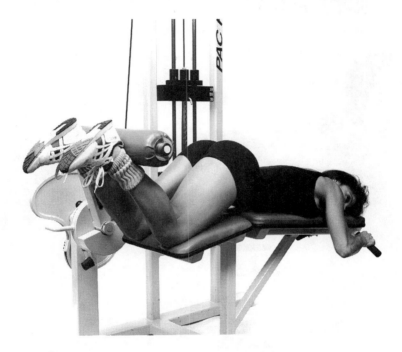

Position yourself so that the pad rests right above the ankle. Bring the pad up to your butt and keep your toes pointed toward the ceiling.

HAMS [Advanced]: Hyperextensions

If you are considerably overweight, don't even think about this very advanced movement, for it will hurt the lower back.

- Lie face down on the hyperextension apparatus, with your hands crossed in front of your chest and the back of your feet pushed against the pad.

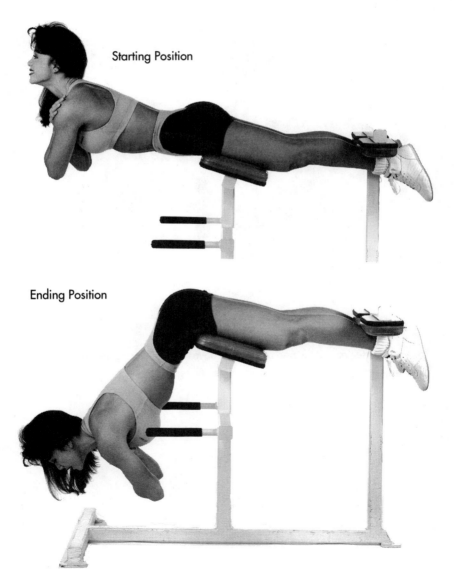

Starting Position

Ending Position

- Relax, drop forward and concentrate on stretching the hamstrings. You don't need to come up high—bring your shoulders up only so they are parallel to the ground.

- If you go any higher, you put undue stress on the spine. This movement should be performed twice as slowly as other movements.

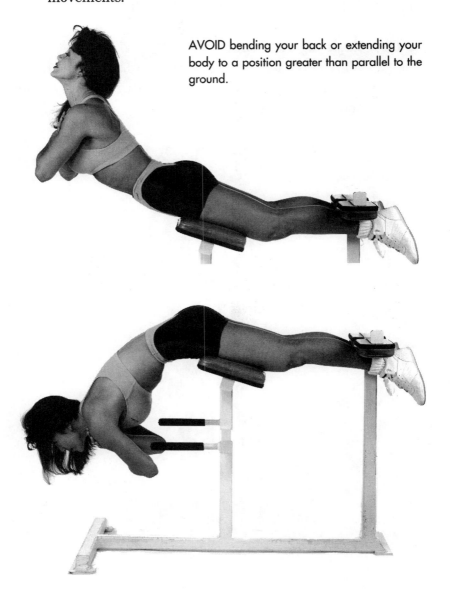

AVOID bending your back or extending your body to a position greater than parallel to the ground.

Calves

Your calves comprise a stubborn muscle group that doesn't re-spond to training as easily as other body parts. Therefore, they get neglected. But they are, if developed, a great body part. Any time you wear shorts or a dress, you can't hide them. A person with developed, nicely toned calves is considered to have good legs, no matter what the rest of his or her legs looks like.

CALVES: Single-Leg Calf Raises

- Standing either on a stair step or even flat on the ground, using either a wall or a chair for balance, wrap one leg gently around the other at the heel.

Starting Position

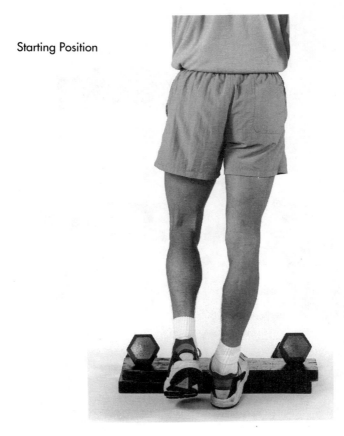

- Then put the weight of your body on the ball of the sole foot that's on the floor and raise up as high as you can go, like a ballerina.

- Then slowly drop down, but without ever letting your wrap-around heel touch the ground. Repeat, then switch legs.

Ending Position

Ending Position—Side View

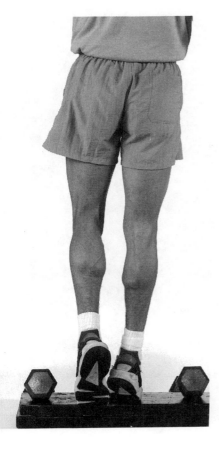

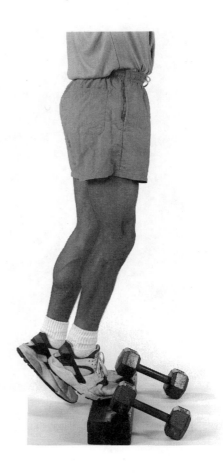

Perform slowly, and concentrate on good posture and a full range of motion.

CALVES [Gym]: Standing Calf Raises

- Using a standing calf raise machine, put your feet on the base of the platform where the heels are off the platform. Keep your feet about four to six inches apart, toes pointed just slightly inward.

- Push up as high as you can go on your toes, and relax as you drop down. Let the heels relax and stretch—and repeat.

Starting Position   Ending Position

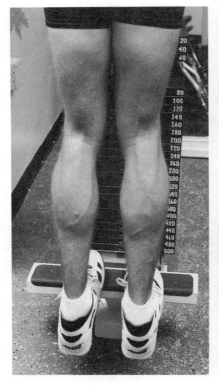 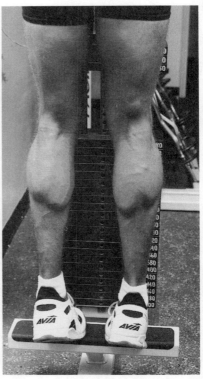

Keep pressure on the balls of the feet. AVOID having the legs locked out, but keep stationary.

CALVES [Advanced]: Seated Calf Raises

- Using a seated calf machine, you perform this the same way as the standing calf raise, only you're sitting down. Standing calf raises work the pretty part of the calf, the seated calf raise works the area of the calf underneath the pretty part.

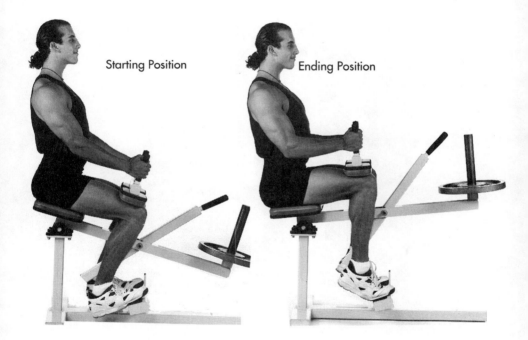

Starting Position   Ending Position

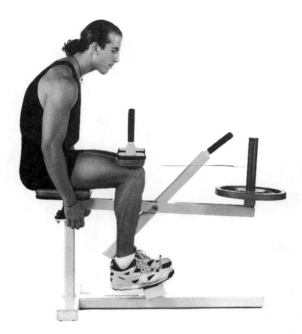

Concentrate on proper posture and foot position. AVOID performing this exercise too rapidly.

Abs

If you have a big belly and you're thinking a lot of abdominal exercises will reduce your waistline, forget about it. Sit-ups do not burn fat; there is no such thing as spot reducing. There was a study done in which a group of people did five thousand sit-ups over a period of twenty-seven days. The study found that there was no difference between the fat lost in the stomach as compared to any other part of the body.

But I'm not knocking your attempts to tighten your ab muscles. As you start to develop your body, the abs are like the focus point of a beautiful picture. The eyes are always drawn to the midsection when looking at a body. So abs will help you complete the entire package. While some experts say you need to train the abs every day, in this program you only need to work them two to three times a week. I want to make sure you work your ab muscles like other muscle groups; perform slowly and contract them tightly and keep so concentrated that you can't perform more than twenty to twenty-five repetitions of each exercise.

If you can do more than twenty-five reps, you're not concentrating hard enough. But when working abs, I want you to develop a rhythm which has you resting very little in between each set and each exercise, much less than with the other movements—anywhere from ten to fifteen seconds per set. Why? We're not using any weight with abs, so you should be able to recover more quickly from each set.

ABS: Crunches

This is the number one exercise for working the abs—not traditional sit-ups, which can hurt your back.

- Lie flat on your back with your legs propped over a bench or chair. Cross your hands over your body (putting your hands behind your head tends to put too much strain on the neck).

- Keep the chin tucked forward into your chest. Come up, just enough to contract the chest.

Starting Position

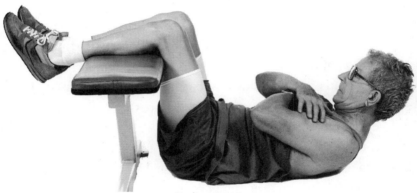

Ending Position

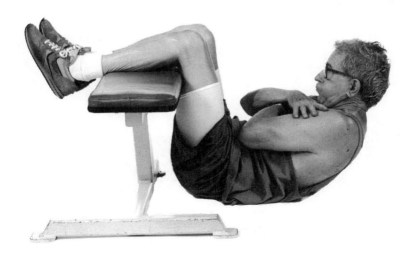

- Now, instead of keeping the upper back straight, you want to curve and roll into the movement. Keep the shoulders round. Always keep your tailbone and lower back on the ground, even when you lift up.

- It's also important to let the air out of your diaphragm at the very beginning as you crunch forward. And as you start the movement, tighten the stomach muscles.

- As you become advanced, you can gradually raise your feet off the bench, holding them a few inches in the air.

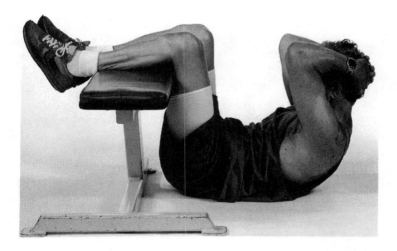

AVOID putting your hands behind your head when doing this exercise. Concentrate on exhaling during exertion.

ABS [Gym]: Hanging Leg Raises

These can be performed on either a hanging leg apparatus or from a chin-up bar, either holding the bar or using arm-support straps.

- Raise your bent knees upwards toward the chest and then come right back down. Don't swing as if you were on a swing set.

Starting Position   Ending Position

- Try not to let your heels ever go behind the body; just lift the knees upward. For beginners, you might want to do one leg at a time.

Ending Position—Front View

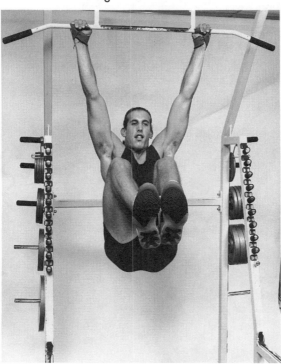

AVOID the tendency to swing. Also, AVOID performing this exercise with your legs straight.

ABS [Advanced]: Jackknife Sit-ups

- Sit at the end of a flat bench. Put your hands behind you on the bench, close to your buttocks, for balance.

- Bend the knees to meet the chest, and at the same time bring the chest to meet the knees. The two should meet in the middle of the movement.

- For the beginner, keep the leg pointed closer to the ground. As you develop more strength in the midsection, keep raising the legs.

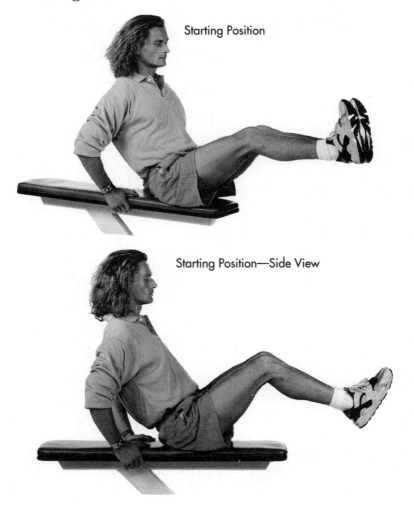

Starting Position

Starting Position—Side View

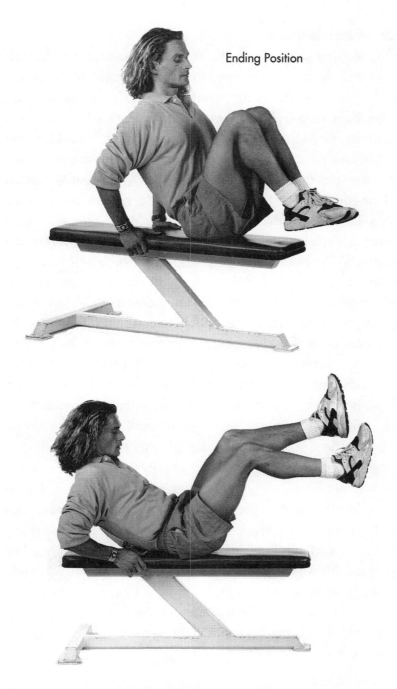

Ending Position

DO keep your legs straight. AVOID leaning too far back.

Order of Muscle Groups

One final thing about your initial training. You want to train your largest muscle groups first, and then go to the smaller muscles. The reason is that small body parts are weak links to larger muscle groups. For example, if you work your shoulders before you work your chest and back, you will be so fatigued in your shoulders you won't be able to get the most out of the chest and back exercises.

So, if you are working on your upper body, you should start off with the chest, then to the back, then shoulders, then triceps, then biceps. There is one exception to this rule. Much later, as you get advanced, if you have a poorly developed body part, or a body part that doesn't respond well to training, work that one first. Why? Because you expend the most energy at the beginning of your workout and you want to have the most intensity focused on the areas of your body that are the most important to you.

I recommend that men begin their workouts on their upper-body parts, then move to their lower body. The reason is that the lower-body parts usually take up so much energy that when men are finished with the lower body, they are often too tired to finish their upper-body workout. But I recommend women begin with lower body because that is generally a higher priority muscle area for them. So if you wish, focus your energy there first.

A word of caution: In the very beginning of your training, for the first two or three weeks, you will feel that all upper-body exercises are affecting only your arms. You might not feel the chest working, or the back working. But you'll always feel the arms working. The reason for this is that your arms are volunteering to do the work. Your body is not accustomed to working your chest and back. So at the beginning of weight training, it's going to feel like arms, arms, arms. Don't worry about it. In time, the proper muscles will do the work.

The Full Body Routine

Want to go for a big workout? Once you're accustomed to all the equipment and once you know your form is right, then try this great full-body routine. You can do it at home or at a gym. Even though it's designed for beginners, you can do this routine forever and continue to improve your body. For each exercise I'm going to give you, do three sets at ten reps each.

1. Incline Barbell Press (for your chest)
2. Flat Bench Flies (chest)
3. One-Arm Dumbbell Row (back)
4. Bent-Over Row (back)
5. Upright Row (shoulders)
6. Side Lateral Raises (shoulders)
7. Lying Triceps Extensions (triceps)
8. Straight Bar Curls (biceps)
9. Lunges (quads and glutes)
10. Front Squats (quads and glutes)
11. Straight-Leg Deadlifts (hams)
12. Single-Leg Calf Raises (calves)
13. Crunches (abs)

Stretching

One of the best ways to avoid soreness or injury is to do some basic stretching exercises at the end of a workout. In fact, stretching can be as important as lifting weights when you're first starting out. You must stretch to avoid the contracted, muscle-bound look. You want to look supple. You want to elongate your muscle. And that's only going to happen if you keep stretching your muscles.

With the right stretching exercises, you are giving your muscles a chance to relax. You are releasing tension out of your body. Moreover, stretching will help shape your body. Your posture will improve. Your body will gain greater mobility and flexibility. Instead of being the kind of weightlifter who can't bend over and touch his toes, you will be lengthening your muscles. You will be creating a beautifully lean, limber appearance.

You can pick from a variety of stretching movements. With the assistance of professional dance instructor and choreographer Gayle Ziaks Halperin, who's also an assistant professor of dance at Texas Women's University in Denton, Texas, I've come up with a routine of stretches that are perfect for weight trainers. Keep in mind there's never a bad time to stretch, only a better time. Stretching best serves its purpose when done *after* the workout or even during a workout.

However, if you want to stretch before a workout, take a long hot shower, which will elevate your body temperature and warm up your muscles. Do not ever stretch cold muscles. If you do, you run the risk of tearing muscle fibers.

Always remember: Do your stretches smoothly. Never bounce when stretching. Never allow your stretching to make your body hurt. Pain is not gain. If you can't touch your toes in a stretch, that's fine. Stretch as far as you can and, eventually, the muscle fibers will lengthen even more. And most importantly, remember to breathe while you are stretching.

Deeply inhale and exhale as you stretch in each position. Hold each stretch for at least twenty seconds, which is approximately four sets of inhales and exhales. Count to three as you inhale and exhale. After getting the hang of the time interval, you will not even have to count. As you inhale, think of relaxing the muscle group, and as you exhale think of elongating the muscle area. Breathing is real important because it uses a natural body rhythm to stretch muscles like elastic bands. If you try to just pull and pull a muscle, it will only give so much. Releasing and relaxing in between will deepen the stretch.

Full Body Stretch

- Put your hands together and then bring them straight up above your head. Hold for twenty seconds. Then gently lower your arms. Think of stretching your hands as far away from your feet as you can. You are trying to lengthen the spine vertically. For the stretch to be effective, form is very important. You don't want to stick your chest out, and you don't want to lower or raise your chin at any time. Nor do you want to suck in your stomach while doing the stretch; instead, think of your navel as touching your spine. This will help make your abdominals work more effectively.

Gayle Ziaks Halperin

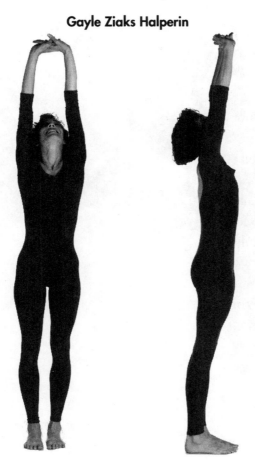

Neck Stretch

- Put the palm of your hand on top of your head and gently bend your head forward. Breathe and hold the stretch for twenty seconds.

- Return your head to its natural position, and then put your right hand on the left side of your head and gently pull your head to the right shoulder. Your ear should be parallel to your shoulder, but not touching it. Then sense the stretch along the left side of your neck and hold as you breathe.

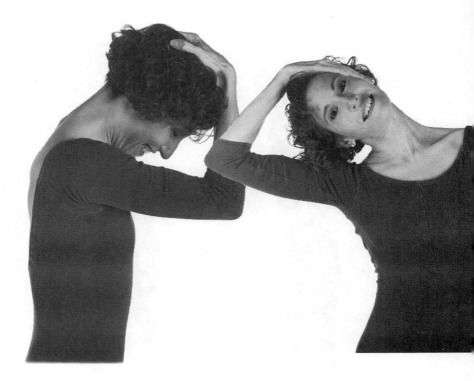

- Return your head to its natural position and switch hands, and do this to the opposite side. This is a simple, but important kind of stretch because in weightlifting, you unconsciously put a lot of tension on the neck, and this stretch will help you release the tightness.

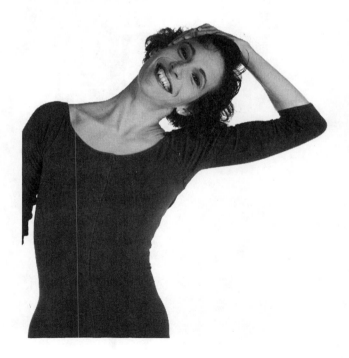

Shoulder Stretch

- Simply inhale and raise your shoulders to your ears—then breathe out and drop your shoulders.

- Also do simple shoulder rolls, circling your shoulders forward and then back around.

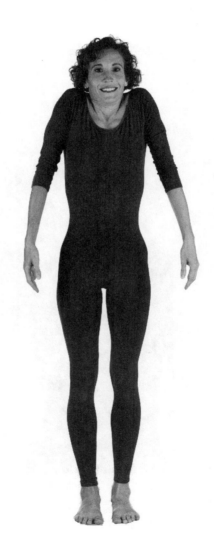

Pectorals Stretch

- Stand directly facing the wall, an arm's length away. Put your arm at shoulder level against the wall, press your hand against the wall and move the body around, shifting your feet in little steps, until you can't go any farther. Hold for twenty seconds. Keep the arm extended, but don't lock the elbows.

- Walk yourself back around to the starting position. Repeat with the other arm. You'll feel a great stretch right across the chest, plus you'll get a partial deltoid and biceps stretch.

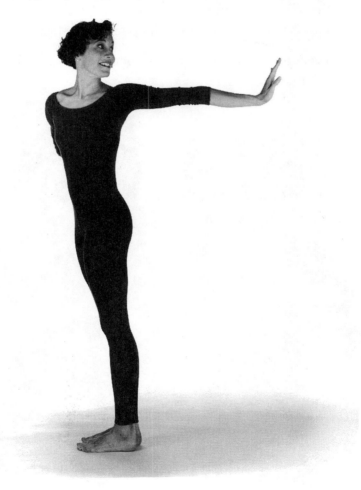

Biceps-Triceps Stretch

- Take your right arm and put it behind your head and it should just about touch the bottom of your neck.

- Put your left hand directly behind your back (right around the waist area) and reach your left hand to the area between the shoulder blades, or as far as you can go. As you stretch, think of lengthening the triceps of the right arm and the biceps of the left arm. Your ultimate objective is to strive to touch the fingertips of both hands. The hands will almost meet between the shoulder blades. Don't force it if you can't touch them together. You're already getting plenty of stretch.

- Breathe and hold for twenty seconds, and then reverse to the other side.

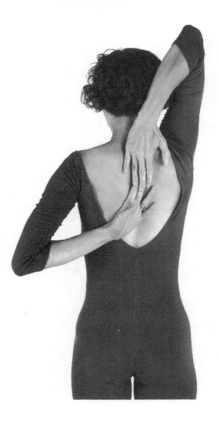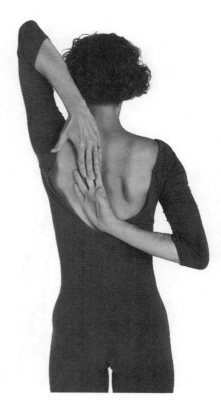

Deltoids Stretch

- Take your right arm across the front of your body until your right arm is beyond your left shoulder.

- Put your left hand under your right shoulder and hold your shoulder.

- Gently pull your right shoulder across the body with your left hand for twenty seconds. Remember to breathe and switch hands for the other side.

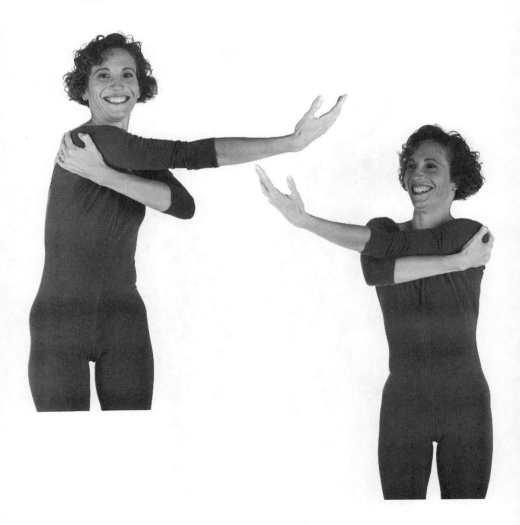

Side Stretch

- Standing with your feet at shoulder-width apart, raise your left arm over your head and then bend your body to the right side. Think of extending your body out into space. Don't contract the right side of your body, but think of lengthening both sides as long as you can.

- Breathe and stretch for twenty seconds.

- Return and reverse to other side.

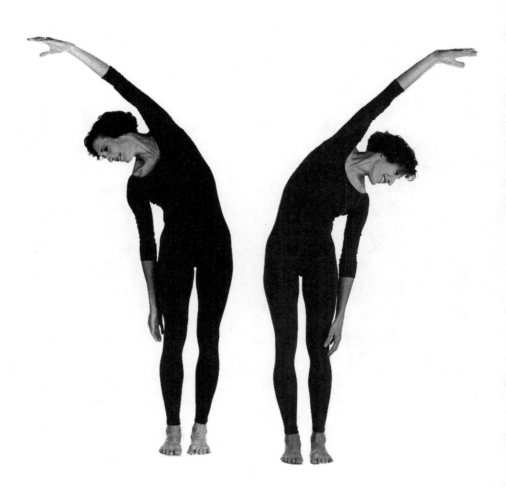

Lower Back Stretch

- Lie on your back with both feet on the floor, your knees sticking straight up.

- Bring the right knee up until it is resting on your body.

- Put your hands below the kneecap and inhale deeply.

- As you exhale, gently pull the right leg closer to your body. As you inhale, allow the right leg to return to its resting position on your chest. Repeat four times. Think of lengthening your lower back as you deepen the flexion of your right hip socket.

- Return the right leg to the floor and reverse to the other side. This stretch is great for anyone with back pain, especially sciatic problems.

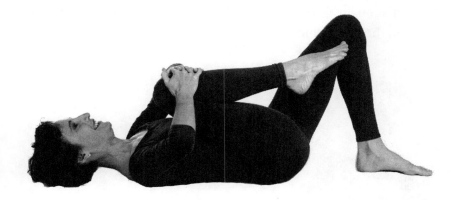

Hips and Gluteus Stretch

Because many people—men, especially—need to stretch their backs, add a second back stretch.

- While lying on your back, fold your left leg into your chest while keeping your right leg long below you.

- Put your right hand below your left knee and then gently bring the left leg across your body past the right leg. This action will force you to somewhat roll onto your right side. However, make sure that both shoulders remain on the floor as you roll because the tendency is to let the left shoulder come off the floor. It is okay if the right leg bends as you stretch the left leg across your body.

- Inhale and as you exhale, gently pull the left leg across the body. Think of relaxing and lengthening the lower back and buttocks. You should feel a stretch from your right hip socket diagonally through your body up to your left shoulder. Repeat to the other side.

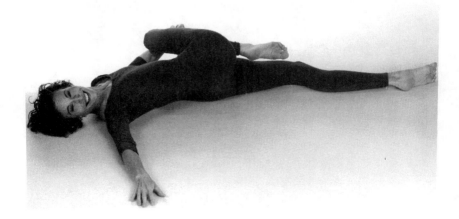

Quadriceps Stretch

- Lie on your back with your feet flat on the floor. Knees are pointing straight up; arms resting across your chest.

- Begin at your tailbone and tilt your pelvis up off the floor. Continue to lift the spine off the floor and stop when you get to your shoulder girdle. You should feel like a bridge. Breathe and stretch for twenty seconds. Feel the quadriceps lengthening away from your hips.

- Then slowly, beginning at the top, lower your spine gently to the floor. Repeat two times.

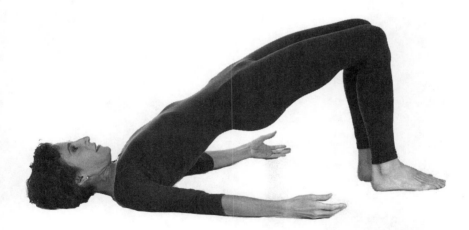

Quadriceps Stretch

- While standing with your feet directly below you, bend your body and legs until your hands touch the floor in front of your toes.

- Pick up your right heel and slide your right leg straight back on its toes until you feel a stretch in your quads. Don't try to go back too far. You don't need to straighten the right leg for a stretch to occur. Also, remember to keep the heel of the left leg flat on the floor and keep your body weight on the left leg.

- Make sure the left knee points forward at all times to prevent torque. Breathe and hold for twenty seconds. Repeat with other leg.

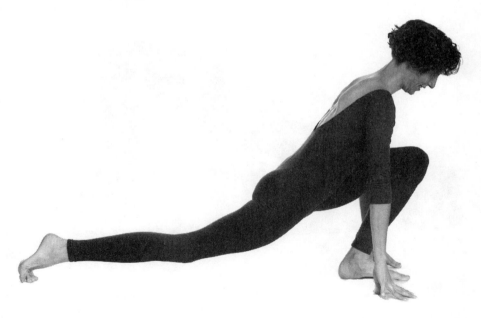

Hamstring Stretch

- Sit on the floor with your legs stretched out directly in front of you.

- Beginning with your head, round your body forward and give in to gravity. If there is tightness, only go as far as you can. Breathe and as you exhale, think of giving in to gravity and of releasing your muscles. It is good to put a rolled towel underneath your kneecaps if you have hyperextended or swayback knees.

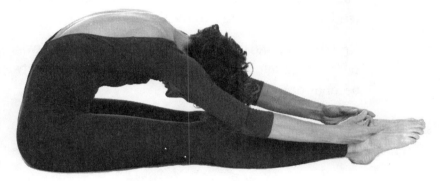

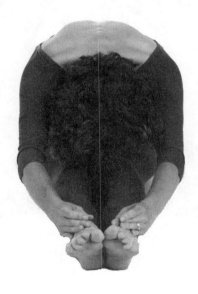

- Open your legs apart to the side just a short distance. It is okay if your legs are bent. If your lower back feels very tight, put a large book, such as the Yellow Pages, under your hips and sit on it. This trick will help release tension and give you elevation allowing you to stretch forward.

- Again, round the spine forward and give in to gravity. Breathe and as you exhale, think of deepening your stretch.

- Twist your body to the right diagonal and bend forward. Keep both hip sockets on the floor because this action has a tendency to lift one hip off the floor.

- Breathe, etc., and then gently return to normal, and twist and bend to the left side. Again, hold every stretch for twenty seconds or more.

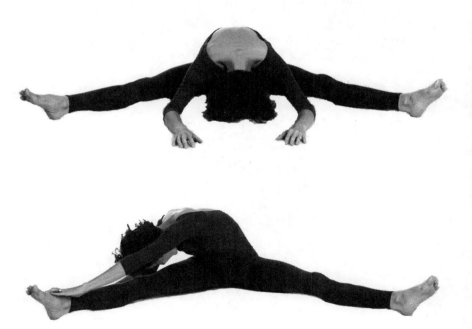

Calf Stretch

- Stand with your feet directly below your hips. Put your palms on a wall directly in front of you. Bend your left leg and slide the right foot back only as far as the heel stays on the floor. This action has caused your body to tilt forward on a diagonal.

- Breathe and as you stretch, think of lengthening the muscles along the back of the lower leg. Again, similar to the quadriceps stretch, make sure the left knee points directly forward and does not lean to the right or left sides, which would produce torque in the kneecap.

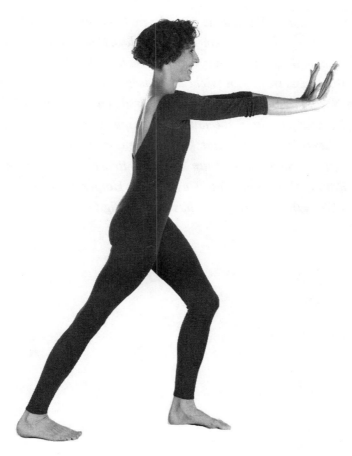

As you do all of these stretches, think of relaxing and releasing muscle tightness through breathing and elongating your muscles. Stretching is enjoyable. If there is pain, ask yourself a few questions: Am I stretching beyond my body's capabilities? Am I trying too hard to touch my toes? How is my form? Am I using my abdominals to provide body stability? Do I need to bend my joints to release stiffness? Am I inhaling and giving in to gravity as I exhale?

After stretching, you should feel longer, taller and broader. And most importantly, you should feel invigorated and refreshed.

Note: Jean Robert Barbette is a model and personal fitness trainer in Aspen, Colorado. He has 5 percent body fat. Jack Heizelman is seventy-five years old with a single-digit body-fat percentage. Adam North is a personal fitness trainer in Wichita, Kansas, with 7 1/2 percent body fat. Alan North has lost more than one hundred pounds of body fat. He is a certified trainer whose specialty is working with overweight people. Reggie Senegal is a world-class, middle-distance runner whose body fat has been measusred at less than 3 percent. Renee Redden was the 1993 Ms. Fitness USA runner-up. Gayle Ziaks Halperin teaches dance at Texas Weslyan University. She has a single-digit body-fat percentage.

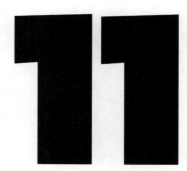

Advanced Weight Training
Improving Your Workouts for an Even Better Body

The body, as you've already been able to tell, adapts to weight training very quickly. Even for those of you who do the most modest routine, your body has no doubt gone through some significant changes. But after your first eight weeks, your body might begin to hit a plateau. A plateau is when you don't feel you're making progress any longer—your muscles don't respond, you're fighting boredom, you seem to be going through the motions. Now is the ideal time to subtly change parts of your routine. Now's the ideal time to make a change.

I'm not talking about anything confusing. You do what you've always done, only this time you want to add in one or more of the following:

1. Increase your number of reps each set. Often, that's all it takes to get that feeling back in your muscles again.

2. Change the order of exercises that you do with your body parts—for instance, do your incline presses after you do flat bench flies. Or, if you're a man, do lower-body exercises before upper body; vice versa for women.

3. Switch to another exercise for that body part. Just look through my various exercises I've already given you, and try something else.

4. Try sitting down for exercises where you normally stand, and standing where you normally sit—but only if the movement

allows you do to this safely. Use an incline or decline bench. Do the exercise standing or sitting. Since your muscles never know what's coming, they're getting challenged.

5. Decrease the amount of time you rest between each set (but never to less than twenty seconds between sets).

6. Only after you've tried everything else should you try to go to heavier weights on each exercise. But make sure your technique remains the number one priority in your weightlifting movements.

Other Plateau Changes

Sometimes, it might not be the weights you need to worry about to break through your plateau. If you are, for example, losing inches but losing strength, then guess what? You're not eating enough. If you aren't putting the right calories into your system, then your body will start getting its nutrients out of the muscle. Eating too little and exercising too much will mean you'll lose lean body mass.

However, if you are getting stronger, but gaining around the waist and around the hips, then guess what? You probably need to shave some food off each meal—and you might need to increase your aerobics to burn more body fat. Remember: your goal is always to lose inches while increasing your strength and having so much energy you barely know what to do with it.

A Split Routine

I also want to introduce you to a routine that I've taught a lot of people in Dallas. It's a three-day-a-week routine that many people follow once they move into the intermediate stages of their training.

On Day One, you train only your upper body. The very next day, Day Two, you train only your lower body. Then you take two complete days of rest. And then, on Day Five, you do a full-body workout. After that, take Days Six and Seven off. And then start all over again.

In this split routine, you are going to be doing an increased amount of work. The reason is that if you train fewer body parts in a single workout—which is what the split routine does—then you need to increase your number of exercises. So here is what you must do: You'll do three exercises (instead of the usual two) on each major muscle group. (You'll keep the same number of two to three sets.) On the smaller muscle groups, you will do two exercises instead of the usual one.

(A quick note to those of you working out at your home gym: If you don't have the machines or the additional equipment needed for the split routine, then simply add sets for your larger muscle groups and smaller muscle groups.) Here's the program:

Day One—Upper Body
You'll do two to three sets, ten reps each.
1. Incline Barbell Presses (chest)
2. Flat Bench Flies (chest)
3. Pec Decks (chest)
4. One-Arm Dumbbell Rows (back)
5. Bent-over Rows (back)
6. Lat Pulldowns (back)
7. Upright Rows (shoulders)
8. Side Lateral Raises (shoulders)
9. Overhead Presses (shoulders)
10. Lying Triceps Extensions (triceps)
11. Push-downs (triceps)
12. Straight Bar Curls (biceps)
13. Incline Dumbbell Curls (biceps)

Day Two—Lower Body
You'll do the same two to three sets per exercise, but you must do twelve to fifteen reps, not ten, because you are doing fewer exercises and you tend to require more reps for your lower body.

1. Lunges (quads and glutes)
2. Front Squats (quads and glutes)
3. Leg Presses (quads and glutes)
4. Straight-Leg Deadlifts (hams)
5. Leg Curls (hams)
6. Single-Leg Calf Raises (calves)
7. Seated Calf Raises (calves)
8. Crunches (abs)
9. Jackknife sit-ups (abs)

Days Three and Four—Rest

Day Five—Full Body

On this day you do your traditional full-body routine that you have already learned. But I want you to increase your repetitions from ten to twelve.

1. Incline Barbell Presses (chest)
2. Flat Bench Flies (chest)
3. One-Arm Dumbbell Rows (back)
4. Bent-over Rows (back)
5. Upright Rows (shoulders)
6. Side Lateral Raises (shoulders)
7. Lying Triceps Extensions (triceps)
8. Straight Bar Curls (biceps)
9. Lunges (quads and glutes)
10. Front Squats (quads and glutes)
11. Straight-Leg Deadlifts (hams)
12. Single-Leg Calf Raises (calves)
13. Crunches (abs)

Days Six and Seven—Rest

The Four-Day Split

If you have really committed yourself to going to the program, and you feel that you need to be in the gym more than three times a week, then you should try the four-day split.

Again, let me make a warning. A four-day routine is the most work you should ever do. Never work more than four days a week unless you're a competitive athlete or bodybuilder. Here's the traditional Four-Day Split:

Day One—Upper Body.

Day Two—Lower Body.

Day Three—Rest.

Day Four—Upper Body.

Day Five—Lower Body.

Day Six and Day Seven—Rest.

The Four-Day Split Routine, Part II

Sometimes during a four-day routine, you should work parts of your lower and upper body on the same day. This constantly challenges the body by giving it something new. What you'll be doing on Day One and Day Three is working your chest, shoulders, triceps and hams and back. On Day Two and Day Four, you'll work your back, biceps, quads and calves. In this routine, we will on occasion increase the number of sets and reps:

Day One

Chest:

1. Incline Presses—three sets, 10-12 reps
2. Dips—three sets, 10 reps
3. Flat Bench Flies—three sets, 12 reps
4. Pec Decks—two sets, 15 reps

Shoulders:

1. Overhead Presses—two to three sets, 12 reps
2. Side Lateral Raises—three sets, 10-12 reps

3. Upright Rows—two to three sets, 8-10 reps

4. Bent-over Lateral Raises—two sets, 12 reps

Triceps:

1. Push-downs—three sets, 12-15 reps

2. Lying Triceps Extensions—four sets, 8-12 reps

Hams:

1. Lying Down Leg Curls—four sets, 12 reps

1. Straight-leg Deadlifts—two to three sets, 10-12 reps

Day Two

Back:

1. Lat Pull-downs (using a wide grip)—three sets, 8-10 reps

2. Bent-over Rows—three sets, 8-10 reps

3. Lat Pull-downs (using a close grip)—two to three sets, 8-12 reps

4. Pull-ups—two to three sets, 6-10 reps

Biceps:

1. Straight Bar Curls—three sets, 10-12 reps

2. Preacher Curls—three to four sets, 10-12 reps

Quads:

1. Leg Extensions—three to four sets, 12-15 reps

2. Leg Presses—three to four sets, 12-20 reps

3. Front Squats—three sets, 12 reps

Calves:

1. Seated Calf Raises—two to three sets, 15-20 reps

2. Standing Calf Raises—two to three sets, 12-15 reps

Day Three—Rest

Day Four—Repeat Day One

Day Five—Repeat Day Two

Days Six and Seven—Rest

For Women Only

I know some of you women are probably still worried that some of these advanced routines are beginning to look too intimidating. You're nervous that you will get too big if you try them. Okay, then here's a great three-day-a-week advanced routine for you that hits on every body part and lets you develop without getting big:

Day One

Chest:
  1. Incline Dumbbell Presses—two to three sets, 10 reps
  2. Pec Decks—two to three sets, 10 reps

Shoulders:
  1. Overhead Presses—two sets, 10 reps
  2. Side Lateral Raises—two sets, 10 reps
  3. Bent-over Lateral Raises—two sets, 10 reps

Triceps:
  1. Push-downs—three sets, 10-12 reps

Legs:
  1. Leg Presses—three sets, 12-15 reps
  2. Hyperextensions—three sets, 12-15 reps
  3. Leg Curls—three sets, 12-15 reps

Day Two

Back:
  1. Lat Pull-downs (using wide grip)—three sets, 10-12 reps
  2. Lat Pull-downs (using close grip)—three sets, 10-12 reps

Biceps:
  1. Curls (using dumbbells or barbell)—three sets, 10-12 reps

Legs:
  1. Leg Extensions—three to four sets, 10-12 reps
  2. Front Squats—three sets, 10-20 reps

3. Larry Lunges—three to four sets, 10-12 each leg
4. Standing Calf Raises—four to five sets, 15-20 reps

Days Three and Four—Rest

Day Five
Legs Only:
1. Leg Extensions—three sets, 10-20 reps
2. Leg Presses—three sets, 10-20 reps
3. Larry Lunges—three sets, 10-20 reps
4. Lying Leg Curls—three sets, 10-20 reps
5. Hyperextensions—three sets, 10-20 reps
6. Seated Calf Raises—three sets, 10-20 reps
7. Standing Calf Raises—three sets, 10-20 reps

Days Six and Seven—Rest

Weak Areas
As you progress, you're going to feel that one body part might not be in shape compared to the rest of your body parts. In that case, you might want to come into the gym and just work that body part. By now, you are knowledgeable enough to pick out any number of exercises that will work your problem area. Here are a few examples to give you an idea:

Better Butt Routine
1. Lying Down Leg Curls—three sets, 12 reps
2. Leg Presses—three sets, 15-20 reps
3. Straight-Leg Dead Lifts—two to three sets, 10-12 reps
4. Hyperextensions—two to three sets, 10-15 reps
5. Larry Lunges—two to three sets, 10 reps (for each leg)

Biceps Blast

1. Straight Bar Curls—three sets, 10 reps
2. Preacher Curls—three sets, 10-12 reps
3. Incline Dumbbell Curls—three sets, 12-15 reps

Head Turner Legs

1. Leg Extensions—three to five sets, 12-15 reps
2. Front Squats—four sets, 20 reps
3. Leg Curls—three sets, 15 reps
4. Straight-Leg Deadlifts—three sets, 12 reps
5. Larry Lunges—five sets, 10 reps
6. Standing Calf Raises—five sets, 12-20 reps

I've Got to Get Big Routine

Don't read this unless you are really advanced and wanting to make your muscles pop out. This routine is for those advanced weight trainers who are dead set on gaining size. It involves five days of training. Each day in the weight room you'll focus on particular body parts, and you'll do lots of sets. On the last training day of the week, you'll do a light upper-body pump, where you reduce the weight and work on the weaker upper-body muscles. It's my favorite routine to increase my strength and build my muscles. You'll see a few new exercises added at the bottom of each day.

Day One

Chest and Front Delts

1. Bench Presses—three to four sets, 8-12 reps
2. Incline Dumbbell Presses—three to four sets, 8-12 reps
3. Dips—three to four sets, 8-12 reps
4. Flies—three to four sets, 8-12 reps
5. Pec Decks—two to three sets, 12-15 reps
6. Front Lateral Raises (like your Side Lateral Raises, only you're raising your dumbbells one at a time in front of you

until they are parallel with your shoulders)—four to five sets, 8-12 reps

Day Two
Back and Traps
1. Pull-ups—three to four sets, 8-10 reps
2. Bent-over Rows—three to four sets, 8-10 reps
3. Lat Pull-downs (wide grip)—three sets, 8-10 reps
4. One-Arm Dumbbell Rows—two sets, 8-10 reps
5. Machine Rows (using the seated row machine for your back, found in weight rooms)—three to four sets, 8-10 reps
6. Shrugs (holding a barbell in front of you, with arms all the way down, move only your shoulders straight up toward your ears)—four to five sets, 8-10 reps

Day Three
Bi's, Tri's and Side Delts
1. Pick any three biceps exercises—three sets, 10-12 reps
2. Pick any three triceps exercises—three sets, 8-12 reps
3. Side Lateral Raises—five sets, 10-12 reps

Day Four
Legs
1. Leg Extensions—three to four sets, 10-20 reps
2. Leg Presses—three sets, 10-20 reps
3. Front Squats—three to four sets, 10-20 reps
4. Larry Lunges—three sets, 10-20 reps
5. Leg Curls—three sets, 10-20 reps
6. Straight-Leg Deadlifts—three sets, 10-20 reps
7. Standing Calf Raises—four sets, 10-20 reps
8. Seated Calf Raises—four sets, 10-20 reps

Day Five—Rest

Day Six

Light Upper Body Pump

1. Flat Bench Flies—three sets, 12 reps
2. Incline Dumbbell Presses—three sets, 12 reps
3. Pec Decks—two sets, 12 reps
4. Pull-Ups—two to three sets, 10 reps
5. Upright Rows—two to three sets, 10 reps
6. Straight Bar Curls—two to four sets, 8-12 reps
7. Incline Dumbbell Curls—two to three sets, 12 reps
8. Triceps Push-downs—three to five sets, 12-15 reps

Day Seven—Rest

One-Body-Part-Per-Day Routine

No matter what I say, there's going to be the die-hard weightlifter who decides to come to the gym every day. All right, if you decide to do it, then try a program where you work out one body part per day. You should do a large number of exercises for that one body part, then leave it alone for a week. For each large muscle, do four to five exercises, going as much as three sets per exercise. For a smaller muscle, do three to four exercises, going two to three sets per exercise. Here's an example:

Day One: Chest—five exercises, three sets each, 8-15 reps per set

Day Two: Back—four to five exercises, three sets, 8-12 reps

Day Three: Shoulders—four exercises, three sets, 8-10 reps

Day Four: Biceps—four exercises, two to three sets, 8-10 reps

Day Five: Triceps—four exercises, two to three sets, 8-15 reps

Day Six: Quads—five exercises, three sets, 8-20 reps

Day Seven: Hams—four exercises, two to three sets, 12-20 reps

Day Eight: Calves—four exercises, two to three sets, 12-20 reps

I do not recommend this as a regular routine, but if you feel you are in a bad plateau and need a change for a week or so, then try it.

Even More Advanced

Once you are fully into the program, far past the beginner's phase, you'll want to try more techniques. What I'm going to show you is not something you should use every workout—not even every other workout. Use them maybe once every four to five workouts.

1. *Forced Reps.* When your muscles wear down during an exercise and you can no longer perform a rep on your own, have someone assist you lifting the weight for one or two additional reps. More than two is a waste of time and can cause injury.

2. *Super Sets.* This is a technique where you do more than one exercise without any rest in between. After a few straight exercises, then you rest. You can super set the same body part—such as flat bench flies with incline presses. Or you can super set unrelated body parts—such as incline presses with lat pull-downs. There's no need to even try super sets for the first three months of your workouts. But later, if you want to increase intensity on the muscles, this is the way to do it.

3. *Training Until Positive Failure.* This is a technique where you start a set and refuse to put the weight down until you can no longer move the weight. This is enormously intense training. Certain people try to do all their training like this—which is nonsense. Your workouts no longer become enjoyable. They become draining and painful and injury-ridden.

4. *Slow Motion Training.* You take two seconds to pull the weight down and four seconds to release it back to the starting position. This is a good technique to teach you to focus on the muscle group you're training. But you don't want to do every single set like this, for it will put too much stress on your joints.

5. *Iso-tension Training.* Here, you squeeze and hold the weight at the top of the movement for a period of time, and then slowly release. An example would be leg extensions, where you hold the weight at the top until you feel a burn, and then let it back down.

6. *Negatives.* This is the technique where you first perform all the repetitions you can complete on your own. Then someone lifts the weight for you for one more rep and you hold it as the weight goes down. On the North Body program, we'll never do negatives. The risk of injury is too great.

Conclusion

It doesn't hurt, as you become advanced, to overhaul your routine every six to twelve weeks, sometimes even going back to a beginning routine for a while. I'd even suggest taking a week off every three months, because you never want to push your body to the point where it simply burns out and becomes liable to get injured.

As much as we've teased the muscle-head mentality of weight rooms, you can actually learn a lot by leafing through muscle and bodybuilding magazines. You'll see a variety of other routines and other movements. Remember: These are routines done by champion bodybuilders who practically live in the weight room and eat up to six thousand calories a day and perhaps use some sort of muscle-inducing drug. If you try to follow these routines, you'll overtrain and burn yourself out. Never make your routine feel like work. If it's not enjoyable, then you need to lighten up.

Sometimes it would benefit you to train with a workout partner. A partner can pay close attention to your routines, correct your form, and motivate you when you feel like leaving the gym. But ultimately, the inspiration must come from within. If you have followed my suggestions through this entire chapter, then think of how far you have already come. Once intimidated by the weight room, you are now a master of it. Once nondescript, your body has begun to develop prized definition. Once flabby, you're now lean.

Now there is only one thing left to do—stick with it. Except perhaps for a book on highly advanced strength training, you will never have to buy another diet or health or fitness book again.

You now have your tools for life.

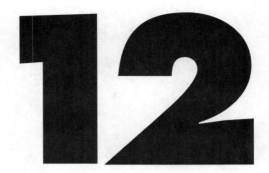

The Second Effort

Building Your
Own Motivation

So here you are, on the next-to-last chapter of this book. At this point, two things should be happening: You should be totally pumped up, leaping for joy that you finally have learned how to break past the old diet and fitness myths. And you still aren't sure you want to embrace a new program. I can hear the comments now, such as:

"I mean, come on Larry, you're not asking me to change just some bad habits. You're asking me to change my life. Larry, the North Program is asking me to give up my 'good life.'"

You have no idea how crazy that sort of comment makes me. I hate fitness people who do a big song and dance about "The New You!" I hate that pitter-patter that says, "Hey, we're going to change your lifestyle!"

I'm not asking you at all to change your life. All I'm asking you to do is change some habits so you can change your body. Period. The North Program is simply a system of replacing bad habits with good ones.

I want you to eat more meals properly, perform longer "true" aerobics, and train with weights three times a week. I want to make you healthier and leaner. This is a lifestyle change? I want you to look more attractive and sexier. This is giving up the good life?

If you think living the good life means having some fantastic cheat meals, fine! This program—as I've said ten thousand times before—is not pass-fail. You can do 50 percent of this program and still be on the program; you'll still see some results. If anything, "the good life," regardless of how you want to define it, will come a lot easier on the North Program, because you'll be living with a fitness program that doesn't torture you or subject you to horrid dieting rules. You won't be punishing yourself with bad workouts. You'll have a life brimming with vast energy.

The Setback

But even as I write this, I know I am not going to reach some of you. I also know that for some of you who have already plunged into the North Program, you're going to back away, at some point in the program, from your commitment to getting lean.

Let's take the example of a woman I know who's really been working out and eating correctly. She's made a lot of progress. Her body is different—shapelier, thinner, more powerful, stunningly attractive—compared to a year ago. People look admiringly at her. She feels a fresh burst of excitement every day. Her life is turning around.

And what does she do? She starts getting off the program! She slows down. She thinks, "Oh, well, there's no way I can go back to the old body. Look how far I've come."

Humans are a strange bunch. Once we get what we want, it seems, we stop wanting it. Moreover, in physical fitness, once we get just close to what we want, we stop wanting it. It's amazing how many people I've watched who make the commitment to get in shape. They get to the crest of the hill. And then, almost without knowing it, they start slacking off. They think they don't have to watch their food consumption as closely. They figure they can miss workouts. They assume it will be easy for them to make a come-back. No, they've had a setback. I've seen people who have gone through fantastic weight loss, whose stomachs have gone from pot bellies to nearly flat bellies. They have had the rare chance, one that only a few people get in life, to develop a great washboard stomach. But then, they stop. Perhaps unconsciously, they have decided that they've had enough.

Learning How to Fight Back

Everyone is going to have setbacks, I know that. I have them, too. And I don't think we should let them upset us, especially the small setbacks. As I've said many times, if you get obsessed over your failures, then you are destined to fail again.

But I know there are a lot of people who just flat-out give up. They work out hard for a year. They take a break. And then they discover that it's even harder to get going again. They relapse again. The process keeps building until these people feel buried by a mountain. They eat poorly for a couple of meals and then decide to go ahead and eat bad the rest of the day. Next, they eat poorly for two days. Soon, their eating program is snowballing out of control.

I know all about people who seem baffled by the possibility of success, who seem far more comfortable with failure. I grew up with a father who was a compulsive gambler. He never worked, never held down a job, but still managed to gamble away thousands of dollars. During his worst phases, he'd steal money out of my mother's pocketbook. He'd pull me out of school to go to the race track with him. We'd spend all day there until he blew his money. Then he'd take me to a fancy restaurant where he'd order a wildly expensive meal. Then, no matter how much money was still in his pocket, he'd walk the check. He'd take me home and then go look for a late-night craps game.

For years I watched him hide from creditors and run from bookmakers who wanted the money he owed them. My father did want to change. He went to Gamblers Anonymous, he went to treatment centers for gamblers. The CBS news show "60 Minutes" did a long story on my father and how he was trying to recover from his gambling addiction.

But the great tragedy of his life—and in my life—was that he never could pick himself back up. He never could fulfill himself as a husband, a father, and a human being. He never knew what it meant to reach his potential. I agonized with him because I loved my father and also because I knew how easy it would be for me, or for anyone, to become like him. As I watched him try and fail, try and fail, over and over, I made a commitment that I would not do the same thing.

If you listen to motivational speakers, they always give you this dreamy picture about how you, too, can be successful. What they never mention is what you must do to get going again once you've had a setback. I learned, through my father, that the key way to stay successful was to learn how to get out of what appeared to be a very small rut. Failure is simply not part of my program.

So, for the final part of this book, you're going to exercise the most valuable, three-pound muscle you have—your brain.

Don't Ever Expect Perfect Progress

What I'm about to say sounds very sacrilegious and un-American compared to the language of every other self-help book that you can read. But if you are looking for immediate results, you're going to fail. The fact is, you can't make permanent changes in your body quickly—and if you'll just recognize that, then you'll take a lot of pressure off yourself.

In the North Program, there's no finish line. What you ultimately want to find most rewarding is the process of getting the North Body—not just the end result. You'll see, from the moment you start, plenty of great results. But just don't ever expect to get to a place where you can say, "I'm finished."

If you do, you'll have a setback. Everyone on his or her eating program is going to go through a process of weight loss, then weight gain, then loss and gain again. Everyone is going to think his or her muscles are, after a period of growth, getting stagnant. But if you conclude, "Well, that's maybe as far as I can go," then you'll hit bottom again.

Talk to people who have been long-time adherents of the North Program. They will tell you that if you keep working out and keep eating properly that the progress will come. They actually stop worrying about tangible progress, whether their waist has gone in an inch or whether they've lost a pound. They know their bodies are always getting better.

Don't Get Down on Yourself

If you study yourself too hard, you'll always find something you did wrong. You'll always be able to say you didn't work out hard enough the previous day or you shouldn't have eaten that one Oreo cookie you saw in the office kitchen. With that kind of attitude, you'll quit pretty quickly. It's hard to stay motivated when you're down on yourself.

If you miss workouts, don't feel guilt-ridden. Don't think you need to run an extra mile or lift weights for thirty extra minutes. This will surely make you hate exercise, because you're turning your workouts into punishment. If you eat a group of cheat meals, don't make the mistake of thinking you need to cut way back on your meals for the next couple of days. Just start back on the program at the next meal. Go to the grocery store and shop for the right foods. Plan your menus very specifically for the day, write them down, and study them—that way you won't deviate. Make sure your refrigerator has plenty of nonfat snack foods like carrots.

Your fitness depends on the everyday personal steps you take today and tomorrow—it does not depend on doing anything drastic. Here's a tip: Instead of visualizing yourself at your worst, visualize yourself at your best. If you hold in your consciousness an image of your body as you wish it to be, then you will want to stick with the program. A real key to this program, oddly enough, is learning how to do "mind workouts." Although you are going to be in a gym which has mirrors covering the walls, you should try to train your mind to forget about a certain part of yourself. As you do this program, you have to forget about your bodily imperfections; you have to forget about what other people in the gym might be thinking about you. You want to focus purely on the joy of doing the program.

When you do that, you've really put out of your mind the possibility of failure.

Too Tired to Get Back into the Gym?

At some point, you're going to look up from your work at the end of a day and say, "I'm just too exhausted to work out."

Don't forget my earlier lesson: Your body gets more energy from a workout than it does if you go home and take a nap.

That still doesn't matter to you? You are still too tired? All right, try this: Do ten quick push-ups on your office floor. Or, sitting on your chair, hold the back of the chair seat with your hands and raise your legs off the floor, bringing your knees to your waist, all the while keeping your back straight.

Not much of a workout, you say? No, it isn't. But it will trigger a kind of muscle memory about how good it feels to work out. Your heart will pump more. You'll get that quick rush that comes from exercise. And you might just say, "You know, working out could make me feel a lot better." You might drop to the floor and do another set of push-ups. You might want to put on tennis shoes and take a walk outside. Or you might head straight to the gym.

When I am feeling listless, I still go to the gym—but I do a very light workout. I don't try to kill myself. I'll walk on the treadmill or I'll do a light, fifteen minute weight routine. Of course, usually after that fifteen minutes, I'm saying, "Hey, I feel pretty good. Let's go another fifteen minutes." Try it. The longer you stay out of the gym, the harder it is to return.

No Time to Get to the Gym?

Ah, here is the greatest excuse of them all. "I've got no time, Larry, just no time." I know you work hard and can't always control your schedule. On Monday, for example, you have to work longer because it's the start of the week or you're on a big project and you're too busy to take an hour in the afternoon to get to the gym. On Tuesday, the same thing happens. It happens again Wednesday. By Thursday, you're getting worn down and you're still busy. That's when you start rationalizing. You'll say, "Well, I blew my workouts for that week. I'll wait until Monday and just start over."

I simply can't believe that you can't find thirty minutes somewhere to work out. If you have time to eat, you have time to work out. In fact, if you make time to work out, you'll ultimately have more time on your hands.

The basic lesson of exercise, as I've said and said and said, is that you develop more vitality. You can concentrate more easily throughout the day. You'll be able to accomplish more things. You'll be able to perform more tasks in an eight-hour day than someone who doesn't work out.

In other words, if you work out, you'll have more time on your hands—which means you'll always have time to work out.

Prepare for the Return of Your Bad Habits

Sometimes, when you feel your dedication starting to slip, you need a strategy in place to keep the bad habit from returning. Be realistic about this. You can give yourself great speeches about staying pumped up all day long. But no speech is going to help you every time. Since you know you're going to get into workout ruts, you've got to anticipate breaking them.

I know a guy who, when he feels the rut coming, sends a letter to his own house from his office. The letter says: "Put down the mail and get on the bike." One of the things he knows he does when he gets into a rut is that he grabs his mail, and sits down near the television to read it. Soon, he's got the remote control in his hands and he's watching the news. His letters to himself are a reminder how easy it is to read his mail and watch television while riding his stationary cycle.

Another guy lays out his workout gear by his bed before he goes to sleep. That way, he has no excuse to search through his drawers and closets in the morning. One time, a woman who knew she was in a rut handed me a CD (compact disc) she had just bought of her favorite musical group. "Don't let me have this until I work out three times this week," she said. I put the CD in a cabinet, and a week later, after her three workouts, she got it back.

Don't Try to Do This Alone

One of the ways to avoid a setback if you feel it coming is to get with someone who knows what you're going through. While you are the one who ultimately has to make the changes in your own life, it doesn't hurt to talk about it with someone else. There has got to be someone at the gym who knows exactly what is happening with you. If you had lunch with such a person, I think both of you would be special ordering and making sure you didn't get in any extra fat. The support alone would send you roaring back into your program.

Conclusion

I want briefly to return, if you'll allow me this indulgence, to the story of my father, Irv North. To get gambling money, he committed bank fraud and mail fraud. As part of his sentence, he was sent to a center to get better—but there, he taught five of the people in his therapy group how to swindle banks. During an outpatient day, he took them all to the race track.

My mother was being driven to the brink of suicide. Finally, when I was a teenager, my mother, my younger twin brothers and I said, "That's it, we're leaving." Without telling my father where we were going, we loaded up a car, packed everything we owned, and sneaked away from our New York home, heading West. We ended up in Dallas, Texas, to begin our life again.

My father and I have long since reconciled. But the saga with him taught me a lot of things. Strangely, he taught me persistence. He was deeply dedicated to his life—one that led him to endless failure and self-destruction. I decided I would be equally dedicated to another kind of life that would take me in an opposite, far more rewarding direction. I was committed to keep going, never to stop, regardless of how many obstacles were put in front of me.

You, too, cannot stop. You must constantly keep your momentum going forward. That is a lesson for your life, and it is a similar lesson for your fitness program. While you may cheat at times, while you may suffer setbacks, while you may slow down—never, ever let yourself stop.

My father used to tell me over and over that he had finally turned the corner. He believed it, and I believed it. But then he would fail again. So when you start to feel really confident in your program, when you think you're really getting good, that's when you need to redouble your efforts to stay fit. Your commitment is not going to come out of thin air. Instead, you must master the art of self-motivation. The price of fitness is responsibility.

My younger brother Alan knows this story all too well. His twin brother Adam, dedicated to the North Program, had always been in great shape. But for a few years, Alan went to live in a different city. When he came back to live with me, he weighed 275 pounds. He had completely discarded everything he had ever learned about health and fitness. When he walked off the plane, I was utterly stunned. Prior to his coming, I had promised him a job at the gym. Now, he was a walking commercial for flab.

"Alan," I said, "you've got to make a commitment to the program."

I have to admit: I wondered if he really would do it or whether he would return to his old habits. But for four months, he did everything that I asked of him. He never cheated on his meals. He never missed a workout. In no time at all, the weight began dropping off of him. Now, he has a thirty-inch waist and very little body fat. He looks great. He's one of the most popular and most knowledgeable trainers in the gym. And he got that way by doing no more than what I am asking of you.

I cannot tell you how excited I am that you have finished this book. There is nothing more satisfying to me than seeing people who realize they have found a program that actually works—that actually shapes their bodies. No person can ever truly be successful if he/she does not feel good about himself/herself. Now, you have that chance. Your physical changes will produce emotional changes, and your emotional changes will produce physical changes. Your new body is going to give you a joy you haven't known before. You'll be more dynamic with people, you'll feel better at work and at home. People will want to look at you; they'll want to be around you because you exude an energy and attractiveness that is rare in this world. That very feeling will keep you wildly enthusiastic about the gym and your eating program.

I've said it a thousand times and I will say it again: Any program that you can't do for the rest of your life is not worth doing for a single day. For as long as you live, you'll have the North Program. All you must do is keep believing in yourself.

I wish you the very best in your journey.

13

Larry North Program Summarized

Never forget that the North Program boils down to some basic principles, which you need to review over and over. So, during those days you need a refresher course, read this handy review:

1. There are no such things as shortcuts to a great body. It is imperative that you find a program that you can do every day of your life. That means you are going to have to get rid of your old notions about food and fitness. Diets are self-destructive and might actually cause you to gain even more weight. Punishing workouts will only harm the body rather than improve it. What you need is a program that offers permanent answers, not another secret formula.

2. To change your body, you've got to give it muscle; not the big, vein-popping muscle you see in bodybuilding magazines, but the pure, lean muscle that contours and shapes the body. To get there, you are going to have to increase your body's metabolism; you've got to speed up the way the body burns fuel. You must take in the right kind of fuel (food) that helps you build your muscle and starve your fat. And you must begin an exercise program that can add muscle to your body. That means only one thing: a weight-training program.

3. Instead of laboriously counting fat grams and calories, concentrate on keeping as much fat and sugar as possible out of

your diet. You want a balance of foods from three food groups: (1) lean protein—which includes white turkey, white chicken, egg whites and the leanest cuts of red meat; (2) complex carbohydrates—which include brown rice, potatoes, oatmeal, whole-grain breads, beans and peas; and (3) fibrous vegetables—which include broccoli, cauliflower, asparagus, spinach, etc. If your eating program consists of one serving each of a lean protein, a complex carbohydrate and a fibrous vegetable (and you can also occasionally throw in a piece of fruit), you'll get so lean your head will spin.

4. When trying to eliminate fat from your diet, all you need to do is eliminate any food containing an abundance of oil, any food high in sugar, and processed foods, and dairy products and any high-fat natural foods such as avocados, olives, nuts and seeds.

5. Instead of eating three huge meals a day, you need to break your eating down into five or six small meals a day. Eating more times throughout the day keeps your body from feeling starved (which, in turn, leads to overeating). Eating more meals also ironically decreases your body's ability to store fat (because you won't be eating big meals that swamp the digestive system). Furthermore, the more you wait between meals, the slower your body's metabolism gets. Smaller, more frequent meals actually increases your body's metabolism, which helps you lose fat.

6. You need a program of true aerobics that does not require profuse sweating and exertion. You need an aerobics program that is low in intensity and long in duration. When you keep your body in motion for a very long period of time and when you don't overexert yourself, you're going to burn off fat. Three to five times a week, for thirty to sixty minutes a session, you need to do a moderate walking, running, swimming or cycling program.

7. The fountain of youth is in the weight room. That's where, with even a light weight-training program, you can totally reshape your body. Always remember: Your form is more important than the amount of weight you use. You must use full range of movement in your arms and legs, and do not exercise halfway. And you never need to do a weight workout that lasts longer than sixty minutes, and never more than three times a week.

8. When you're lagging—going back to your old eating habits or missing workouts—don't get down on yourself. Don't feel a need to punish yourself with an extra-long workout. Go into the weight room and do a light routine. Make yourself enjoy working out again. Plan your menus very carefully. Write down exactly what you want to eat for that day at each meal. Keep the list with you. Most importantly, do a "mental workout," where you visualize yourself in peak condition. That should inspire you enough to avoid any major setback.

Appendix

Bodybuilder Muffins
Preheat oven to 375 degrees

Ingredients:
2 cups rolled oats
10 egg whites (about 1 ¹/₂ cups)
2 Granny Smith apples, chopped
1 tsp. cinnamon
¹/₂ tsp. vanilla
3 pkg. Sweet and Low (not Equal), or 3 tsp. honey
1 tsp. grated orange/lemon zest, optional
¹/₂ cup raisins, optional

Combine all ingredients. Mix with an electric mixer about two minutes. Pour into nonstick muffin pans. Bake in preheated 375-degree oven for 15-20 minutes. Store in ziplocks in refrigerator.

Fake Fried Chicken
(Low-fat chicken), Serves 4
Preheat oven to 350 degrees

Ingredients:
4 boneless, skinless chicken breasts, trimmed of fat
1 cup bread crumbs

1 tsp. garlic powder
1 tsp. Italian herb seasoning
salt and pepper to taste
1 egg white
¹/₂ cup skim milk
a little chicken broth, defatted

Trim all visible fat from chicken. Wash and pat dry. Combine all other ingredients in a gallon ziplock bag. Put chicken in and shake. Beat egg white and milk together in a bowl. Dip breaded chicken in egg mixture. Put chicken back in ziplock and shake again. Place on foil-covered cookie sheet sprayed with nonstick cooking spray. Mist with chicken broth and bake for 20 to 30 minutes in preheated, 350-degree oven.

Enchilada Casserole
(Low fat), Serves 4-6
Preheat oven to 350 degrees

Ingredients:
1 pound ground sirloin or 90 percent lean beef
1 pound macaroni, cooked according to package instructions
1 pound frozen corn, regular or mixed with red and green pepper
One 28-oz. can Progresso tomato sauce
2 cans Rotel tomatoes
1 large onion, chopped
1 green pepper, chopped
2 packages Lawry's taco seasoning
1 tsp. garlic powder
grated nonfat cheddar cheese (optional)

Brown ground meat in skillet. Place browned meat in colander and rinse under hot water to remove any excess fat drippings, drain. In a large saucepan, brown onions and add green peppers. Add ground meat, tomato sauce, tomatoes and seasonings. Cook for about 10 minutes. Add a little water if sauce is too thick. Add corn. Stir to mix. Add macaroni. Place mixture in a large casserole, sprinkle with cheese if desired and bake 20 minutes at 350 degrees or until bubbly.

Note: You may add more corn, fresh tomatoes, picante sauce or jalapeno peppers.

Chicken Flautas
(Low-fat Mexican), Serves 4-6
Preheat oven to 400 degrees

Ingredients:
1 ¹/₂ pounds boneless, skinless chicken breasts, trimmed of all visible fat and sliced in ¹/₂-inch strips
1 large onion, chopped
One 7-oz. can chopped green chilies
1 tsp. garlic powder
1 tsp. ground cumin
¹/₂ tsp. ground oregano
enough chicken broth to cover chicken
1 can Rotel or 1 cup picante sauce
salt, pepper, cayenne pepper and jalapenos to taste
sliced jalapenos and sliced onions for garnish
nonfat white cheese or low-fat Monterey jack for garnish
fresh cilantro for garnish
white corn tortillas

Place chicken in a pan with enough broth to cover it. Bring chicken to a boil, lower heat, simmer gently approximately 30 minutes. Mash up the chicken, add the onions, chilies, rotel and seasonings, and continue to cook until most of the broth is absorbed. Dampen corn tortillas with water, heat in the microwave 30 seconds to 1 minute until soft. Put a couple of tablespoons of the chicken